CLEANLINESS IS NEXT TO GODLINESS

Studies in Australasian Historical Archaeology

Martin Gibbs and Mary Casey, Series Editors

The Studies in Australasian Historical Archaeology series aims to publish excavation reports and regional syntheses that deal with research into the historical archaeology of Australia, New Zealand and the Asia-Pacific region. The series aims to encourage greater public access to the results of major research and consultancy investigations, and it is co-published with the Australasian Society for Historical Archaeology.

An archaeology of institutional confinement: the Hyde Park Barracks, 1848–1886
Peter Davies, Penny Crook and Tim Murray

Archaeology and history of the Chinese in southern New Zealand during the nineteenth century: a study of acculturation, adaptation and change
Neville A. Ritchie

Archaeology of the Chinese fishing industry in colonial Victoria
Alister M. Bowen

Cleanliness is next to godliness: an archaeological perspective on the influences of Victorian values and city-wide health in Parramatta, New South Wales
E. Jeanne Harris

The commonwealth block, Melbourne: a historical archaeology
Tim Murray, Kristal Buckley, Sarah Hayes, Geoff Hewitt, Justin McCarthy, Richard Mackay, Barbara Minchinton, Charlotte Smith, Jeremy Smith and Bronwyn Woff

Flashy, fun and functional: how things helped to invent Melbourne's gold rush mayor
Sarah Hayes

Good taste, fashion, luxury: a genteel Melbourne family and their rubbish
Sarah Hayes

Port Essington: the historical archaeology of a north Australian nineteenth-century military outpost
Jim Allen

Recovering convict lives: a historical archaeology of the Port Arthur penitentiary
Richard Tuffin, David Roe, Sylvana Szydzik, E. Jeanne Harris and Ashley Matic

The shore whalers of Western Australia: historical archaeology of a maritime frontier
Martin Gibbs

CLEANLINESS IS NEXT TO GODLINESS

An archaeological perspective on the influences
of Victorian values and city-wide health
in Parramatta, New South Wales

E. Jeanne Harris

Studies in Australasian Historical Archaeology
Volume 10

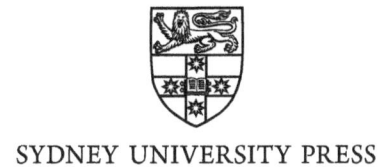

SYDNEY UNIVERSITY PRESS

Published 2025 by Sydney University Press
In association with the Australasian Society for Historical Archaeology
asha.org.au

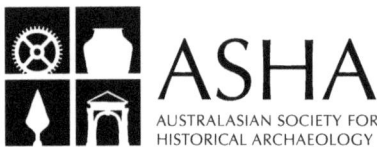

© E. Jeanne Harris 2025
© Sydney University Press 2025

Reproduction and communication for other purposes
Except as permitted under Australia's *Copyright Act 1968*, no part of this edition may be reproduced, stored in a retrieval system, or communicated in any form or by any means without prior written permission. All requests for reproduction or communication should be made to Sydney University Press at the address below:

Sydney University Press
Gadigal Country
Fisher Library F03
University of Sydney NSW 2006
AUSTRALIA
sup.info@sydney.edu.au
sydneyuniversitypress.com

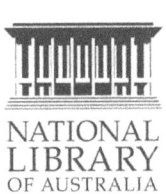 A catalogue record for this book is available from the National Library of Australia.

ISBN 9781761540110 paperback
ISBN 9781761540172 epub
ISBN 9781761540158 pdf

Cover image: Cleanliness is next to godliness. Lithograph by Henry Stacy Marks, approximately 1890.

We acknowledge the traditional owners of the lands on which Sydney University Press is located, the Gadigal people of the Eora Nation, and we pay our respects to the knowledge embedded forever within the Aboriginal Custodianship of Country.

Some quotations from historical sources may contain terms or views that are culturally sensitive, outdated, or discriminatory, and do not reflect current understanding or contemporary values. The wording in these quotes does not reflect the views of Sydney University Press or the author.

CONTENTS

List of figures	vii
List of tables	ix

1. Nineteenth-century health and Victorian values   1
   Australian health and medicine   1
      Parramatta in the long 19th century   4
      Medical anthropology   4
      Organisation of this volume   5

2. Brief history of Parramatta   7
   Time period 1 – convict settlement (1789–1820s)   7
   Time period 2 – Market town (1820–1830s)   9
   Time period 3 – moving forward (1840–1860s)   13
   Time period 4 – feast and famine (1870s–1900)   14
   Time period 5 – a new nation (1901)   15

3. Creating a case study   17
   Case study: city-wide Parramatta   17
      Archaeological site selection criteria   17
      Environmental reforms: public and private health initiatives evidenced in structural remains   18
      Social reforms: evidence of personal health practices in artefact collections   19
   Personal health artefact analysis   19

4. Australian class and social structure   21
   Development of colonial class formation   21
   The making of colonial social structure   22
   Australian class structure   23
   Victorian values and their health implications   25
      Cleanliness   25
      Sobriety   26
      Piety – the role of religion   28
      Work ethic   29
      Chastity   29
   Victorian values in literature   29

5. The archaeology of social class   31
   Establishing social status for the Parramatta case-study households: archaeological evidence   32
   Establishing social status for the Parramatta case-study households: documentary evidence   35

6. The history of colonial medicine, public health and environmental reform   39
   Relevant medical history sources   39
   The language of medical history   39
   Public and personal health   39
   Personal health in 19th-century Australia   41
   Public health and environmental reforms in colonial Parramatta   41
   Colonial public health: historical sources   42
      Nutrition   42
      Institutions of health   45
      Friendly societies   46
      Management of diseases and epidemics   48
   Environmental reforms: multiple lines of evidence   49
      Public and private health initiatives for resolution of Parramatta water issues   53

	The need for clean water supply in Parramatta	56
	Water contamination	56
	Noxious trades	57
	Archaeological evidence of environmental reforms	59
7.	**The archaeology of personal health and social reforms**	**61**
	Traditional medicine and self-medication	61
	Physicians and medical practitioners	62
	Women's health	63
	Consumer choice for self-medication	64
	Parramatta study of patent medicines: archaeological evidence	65
	Mould, water pollution and patent medicines	68
	Personal hygiene and grooming	68
	Ablutions	69
	Oral hygiene	72
	Laundry and household cleanliness	73
	Personal grooming	73
	Vices – patterns of alcohol and tobacco consumption	76
	Alcohol	76
	Archaeological evidence for alcohol consumption	76
	Schnapps	79
	Non-alcoholic beverages: aerated water	81
	Discussion	84
	Tobacco use – health, temperance and social values	85
	Temperance	85
	Archaeological evidence	85
	Discussion	87
8.	**Colonial Parramatta: a medical anthropological approach to health and class**	**89**
	Cleanliness is next to godliness: a primary indicator of respectability and compliance with Victorian values	90
	Environmental reforms for cleanliness	90
	Social reforms	91
	Vices and cleanliness	93
	Attitudes towards medical reform	94
	The science of medical reform	94
	The church and medical reform	95
	The two faces of Australian social class structure	95
	The public face of respectability	95
	The private face of respectability	96
	Discrimination towards the disrespectable	98
	Where they lived	99
	Where they obtained health care	100
Concluding remarks		**101**
Appendix: sites in the case study		**103**
	Site 1: 4 George Street	104
	Site 2: 15 Macquarie Street	106
	Site 3: 45 Macquarie Street	107
	Sites 4–5: Wentworth Estate, 2 and 13–15 Taylor Street	108
	Site 6: 100 George Street	110
	Site 7: 2 George Street	112
	Site 8: 109 George Street	114
References		**115**
	Unpublished source material – reports	122
	Unpublished source material – theses	123
	Internet sources	124
	Newspapers and historical sources	125
Index		**127**

LIST OF FIGURES

Figure 1.1 Location of Parramatta.	2
Figure 2.1 An 1814 plan of Parramatta commissioned by Governor Lachlan Macquarie.	10
Figure 2.2 Sketch of Parramatta, April 1793, by Fernando Brambila, showing the early convict settlement at Parramatta.	10
Figure 2.3 Fleury's 1853 view of the Byrnes Cotton Mill located on the Parramatta River.	12
Figure 2.4 The 1839 Lennox Bridge, spanning the Parramatta River, was photographed around July 1870 by Henry Beaufoy Merlin of the American and Australasian Photographic Company.	13
Figure 6.1 Reconstructed 1800s sketch showing a cottage and garden, Barrack Lane, Parramatta.	43
Figure 6.2 A view showing the first, early 19th-century Government House, Sydney, and its vegetable gardens.	44
Figure 6.3 Plan Map showing Parramatta's structures that were institutions of health.	45
Figure 6.4 A c.1908 view of George Street showing the Parramatta United Friendly Society Medical Institute.	47
Figure 6.5 A 20th-century postcard showing Experiment Farm Cottage.	51
Figure 6.6 A photograph showing Aldine House, Rowland Hassall's home (1804–1882).	52
Figure 6.7 A section of the town drain that crosses 3 Parramatta Square.	53
Figure 6.8 Plan map of Parramatta showing elevation and the course of the Town Drain.	54
Figure 6.9 Howell's 1828 flour mill constructed on the banks of the Parramatta River.	58
Figure 6.10 Sketch showing the 1841 Byrnes Steam Mill.	59
Figure 7.1 Toothbrushes recovered from 4 George Street (site 1).	73
Figure 7.2 Hair combs recovered from 4 George Street (site 1).	74
Figure 7.3 Shaving product tins recovered from 13–15 Taylor Street (site 5).	74
Figure 7.4 Graphic representation of Dingle's per capita annual alcohol consumption for New South Wales.	78
Figure 7.5 Graphic representation of Dingle's per capita alcohol consumption for Great Britain.	79
Figure 8.1 An 1844 sketch of female convicts doing laundry at the Parramatta Female Factory.	92
Figure 8.2 Late 19th century Udolpho Wolfe trade card (with recipes on reverse side).	97
Figure 8.3 View of Parramatta looking towards the Governor's House (1798).	98
Figure 8.4 View of the redoubt at Rose Hill, drawn by E. Dayes from a sketch by J. Hunter.	99
Figure A.1 Plan of Parramatta showing the locations of sites in the case study.	103
Figure A.2 Cesspit at 4 George Street (site 1) that is used in the case study.	105
Figure A.3 Early drain and partially excavated pond at 15 Macquarie Street (site 2).	106
Figure A.4 Well at the rear of 45 Macquarie Street (site 3) that is used in the case-study.	107
Figure A.5 A 1907 Sydney Water map showing semidetached dwellings on the west side of Taylor Street (sites 4–5).	108
Figure A.6 Northern cistern at the rear of 2 Taylor Street (site 4).	109
Figure A.7 Cistern at the rear of 15 Taylor Street (site 5).	109
Figure A.8 Cesspit (site 6). Allotment 70, 100 George Street, used in the case study.	110
Figure A.9 Cesspit (site 6). Allotment 70, 100 George Street, used in the case study.	111
Figure A.10 Well (site 6). Allotment 69, 100 George Street, used in the case study.	111
Figure A.11 An 1804–05 watercolour of convict huts along High Street (now George Street), Parramatta.	112
Figure A.12 Cellar at 2 George Street (site 7), used in the case study.	113
Figure A.13 Cellar profile at 2 George Street (site 7), used in the case study.	113

LIST OF TABLES

Table 2.1 A Timeline of key events in Parramatta's history.	8
Table 2.2 Parramatta Population Chart 1788–1911.	11
Table 5.1 House types identified for case-study sites.	32
Table 5.2 Relative frequencies of European porcelain vessel forms calculated for case-study sites.	33
Table 5.3 Relative frequencies of glass tableware by quality established for case-study sites.	34
Table 5.4 Summary information for the status and class of residents in the case study.	35
Table 5.5 Summary of occupations and activities identified for middle-class residents of Taylor Street.	36
Table 6.1 A list of defined terms used for medical practitioners.	40
Table 6.2 Weekly food rations were provided to all settlers based on the First Fleet Rations.	42
Table 6.3 Dates identified for the development of vaccines for contagions.	48
Table 6.4 Summary showing drainage issues for case-study sites.	55
Table 7.1 Basic contents found in a home medicine chest.	62
Table 7.2 Identified categories of medicine bottles in the 2019 study on patent medicine bottles from Parramatta archaeological sites.	66
Table 7.3 Categories of medical complaints and relative frequencies identified in the 2019 patent medicine study area.	66
Table 7.4 Relative frequencies of medicine bottle types indentified in the 2019 patent medicine study in Parramatta.	67
Table 7.5 Patent medicines from case-study sites used for the treatment of symptoms of environmental contamination.	69
Table 7.6 Patent medicine treatments from case-study sites that were used to combat symptoms of mould and water pollution.	69
Table 7.7 Quantitative data tabulated for personal hygiene-related artefacts ordered by feature dates.	70
Table 7.8 Relative frequencies calculated for personal hygiene artefacts for case-study sites.	71
Table 7.9 Relative frequencies calculated for personal grooming artefacts for case-study sites.	75
Table 7.10 Illustrations, photographs and descriptions of alcohol bottle types identified in the case study.	77
Table 7.11 Relative frequencies calculated for beverage types from features in case-study sites.	80
Table 7.12 Relative frequencies of alcohol and aerated water bottles recovered from case-study sites in chronological order.	82
Table 7.13 Relative frequencies calculated for tobacco pipes from case-study sites in chronological order.	87
Table A.1 Summary information for features at case-study sites.	104
Table A.2. Summary information for features from 100 George Street used in the case study.	110

Chapter 1
NINETEENTH-CENTURY HEALTH AND VICTORIAN VALUES

For more than 30 years, archaeologists have recorded and studied the colonial past of Parramatta, the second-oldest European settlement in New South Wales. Archaeological investigation has provided a wealth of information that contributes to the interpretation of the landscape, the history of the town's development and our knowledge of the people who lived there. *Cleanliness is next to godliness* will use archaeological assemblages generated by these investigations as the basis for exploring what these mainly British settlers and their descendants have as societal beliefs, principles and norms (termed "Victorian values"), which emerged concerning cleanliness and health-related issues. This research is the first scholarly work that presents the archaeology of Victorian social conventions as something more than respectability manifested as socio-economic status, manners and etiquette.

Parramatta is a world-class archaeological site (see Figure 1.1). More than 120 archaeological consultancy reports, as well as numerous journal articles, publications and academic dissertations, provide us with a wealth of data. While many focus on specific sites, others have embraced a city-wide perspective. Examples include Higginbotham's studies of landscape topography and drainage systems, which explored environmental issues faced by Parramatta's early European population, while MacPhail and Casey's investigation of plant microfossils provided insight into their crops and dietary patterns.[1] Parker's work examined the archaeological remains from convict huts to better understand early construction methods using locally sourced materials, and Harris' study of 19th-century medicine bottles illustrated the health concerns faced by Parramatta's residents.[2] While these single-themed studies contribute to our understanding, they are just the first step to addressing how such studies create and overview of Parramatta's history from an archaeological prespective.

Cleanliness is next to godliness demonstrates how, by synthesising this rich body of archaeological resources, we have the opportunity to pursue a city-wide perspective that paints a fuller picture of the day-to-day lives of the people who occupied Parramatta during the long 19th century (1788–early 1900s). It draws on the data from more than 30 studies of Parramatta archaeological sites, 20 Parramatta-specific histories and articles, and contemporary reports contained in more than 20 local and regional newspapers.[3] This information is explored through a framework of medical anthropology, which enables an understanding of the fundamental importance of sociocultural relationships in health and illness. It also draws on a range of other disciplines, including health and medical sciences, as well as an understanding of class structure, commerce and government regulation.

Australian health and medicine

Health is "not merely the absence of disease and infirmity but complete physical, mental and social wellbeing".[4]

Embedded in the 21st-century Australian lifestyle is an ethos to strive for good health.[5] Fresh air, exercise and good personal hygiene are an everyday part of life, as is information on maintaining good health. The sources for such knowledge seem endless, from the food products on shop shelves to literature, media and government educational initiatives. The Australian social structure incorporates medical systems that have evolved over the last two centuries. These systems are not merely the patient's and the practitioner's interaction but rather systems that intertwine with kinship, social values, politics, economy and religion.[6] Evidence that these influences are interwoven with colonial health can be exemplified in the lives of the colony's early residents.

Understanding cultural effects on health is assessed by answering questions such as: What determines health and illness in a culture? How does a society approach its health care system? What role does culture play in the effectiveness of treatments?[7] A culture's conception of health includes its belief that a symptom is or is not indicative of an illness. For example, in late 18th-century Australian culture, the concept of excessive alcohol consumption as an illness did not exist. Imbibing was considered in terms of social conventions, attributing patterns of drinking to social class. Indeed, the term "alcoholism" did not exist until the early 1800s when German physicians constructed a new vocabulary to describe the disease.[8] Therefore, cultural and social views regarding excessive drinking affected attitudes towards this behaviour during those times.

---

1   Higginbotham 2004; MacPhail and Casey 2008.
2   Harris 2019; Parker 2006.
3   Harris 2021, 185–6.
4   World Health Organization 1978.
5   Eckersley 2001, 69.
6   Baer et.al 2003, 9.
7   Singer and Baer 2012, 8.
8   Lewis 1992, 98.

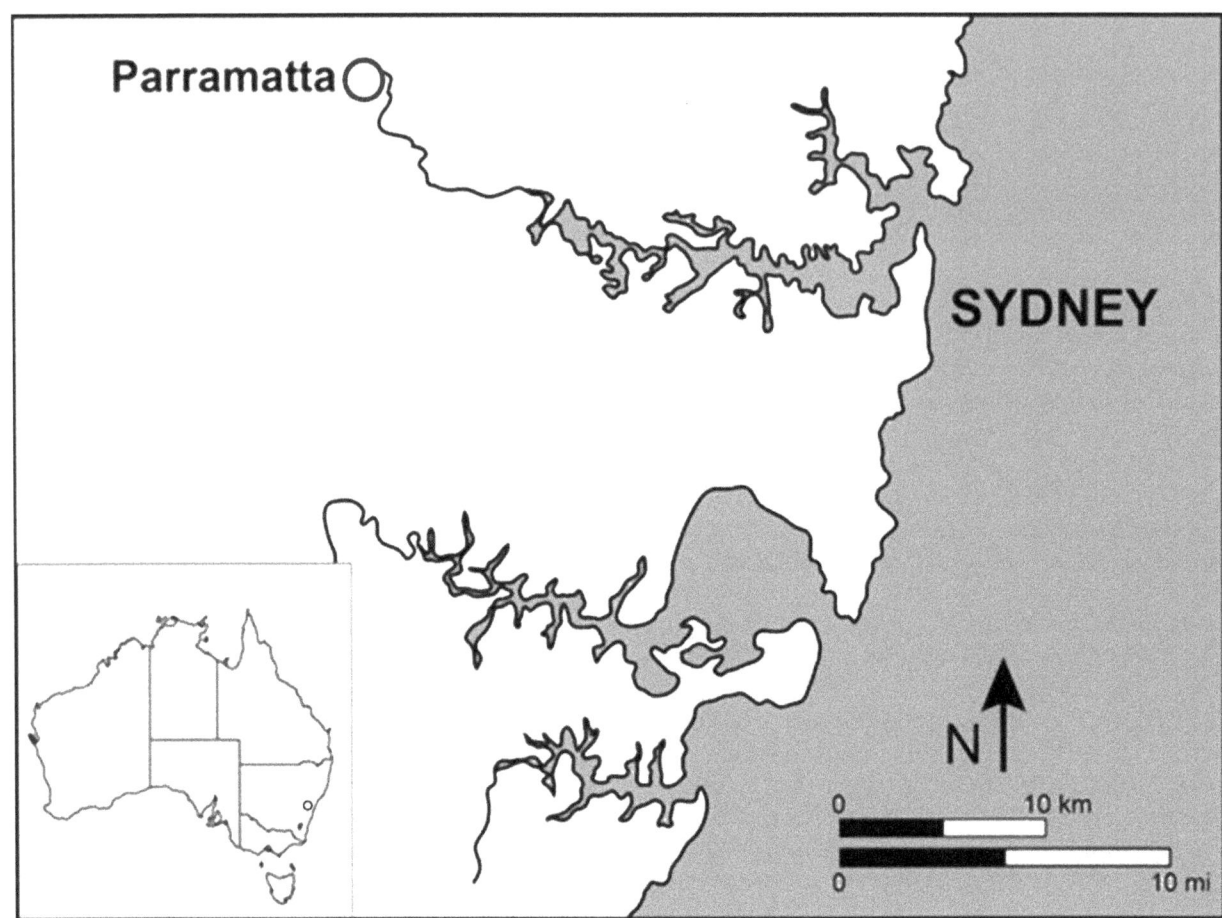

Figure 1.1 Location of Parramatta. Source: E.J. Harris 2017.

As the 19th century progressed, approaches to medicine also changed. During the first 50 years of the colony, medical services for all colonists were provided by the Colonial Medical Service, established by naval surgeons upon the arrival of the First Fleet in 1788 to see to the health of convicts, military personnel and later the free settlers. After 1838 only convicts and the destitute had access to government medical services and the high cost of medical care meant only the wealthy and middle-class settlers could afford to pay for formal health services. This meant that, for the working class, access to medical care was often restricted to home remedies and patent medicines. One such person was Hannah Green. In 1889, when Hannah Green's husband lost his job, they could no longer afford membership fees for the local friendly societies (mutual aid groups) that offered access to an affordable medical dispensary. There were few socially acceptable sources of employment for a mother of four, so Hannah took in washing to support her children. Imagine her distress when she fell pregnant with her fifth child, a child she could not afford to feed, clothe or tend while she continued to be the sole supporter of her family. Seeking to terminate her pregnancy, Mrs Green chose to ingest Beecham's Pills, commonly rumoured to induce a miscarriage,[9] as well as pills of bitter apples and bitter sloes that ultimately resulted in her death.[10] Sadly, Mrs Green was not the only working-class married woman in Parramatta to resort to unorthodox medical methods to induce abortion.[11]

Intertwined in these stories of colonial lives are the social conventions that affected Australia's colonial health: Victorian values that directly and indirectly influenced attitudes towards colonial health. The exploration of the roots and evolution of Victorian social values and how they are demonstrated in the archaeological record can best be achieved through theories based in medical anthropology. The sociocultural factors associated with core Victorian values are just as relevant to health as they are to history, archaeology and medicine. Medical anthropologists define health as not just an absolute state of being, but rather a varying concept depending on the perceptions of sociocultural context. Investigating the sociocultural effects of health in Australia requires understanding the evolution of its society and culture and how it developed in the unique Australian colonial setting.

---

9 Sprenger 2012, 75.

10 *Cootamundra Herald*, 10 April 1889, 3.

11 "Orthodox" (or allopathic) medicine treats symptoms and diseases with prescribed compounds and drugs and invasive surgery.

1 Nineteenth-century health and Victorian values

Surgeon John Irving, who arrived in Parramatta as a convict in 1791, strove to uphold what can be prematurely termed "Victorian values" and through his dedication to his profession became the colony's first emancipated convict. Irving was given a 12-hectare (30-acre) land grant north of Parramatta and had aspirations of starting a new life as a private practitioner and gentleman farmer, allowing him to assimilate into colonial middle-class society. He failed, due in part to his failure to successfully cooperate with the increasingly powerful and corrupt military "Rum Corps" that controlled access to goods such as food, clothing and labour through a complex bartering system using rum as payment. Irving could not afford the exorbitant prices set by those in power and it has been reported that his access to special prices was blocked by his refusal to take up the position of abortionist to cater to the needs of the Rum Corps. For John Irving, unsuccessful attempts to establish his private medical practice and his less-than-mediocre farming success led to him drowning his failures in alcohol. This ultimately led to his death on 3 September 1795 and Parramatta losing a much-needed healthcare provider.

Unlike Irving, Mary Mumford's story is one of eventual success and acceptance. Arriving in the colony as a convict in 1827, 37-year-old Mary was a trained midwife, yet her struggle to succeed in her profession was fraught with social prejudices. Like many female convicts, Mary entered a de facto relationship for social, physical and sexual protection.[12] Despite successfully using her medical skills to aid expectant mothers through the birthing process, her ticket of leave (which gave convicts freedom to work for themselves) was cancelled in 1833 when it was found she was living in a state of prostitution (de facto) with fellow convict Martin Gambell, whom she could not legally marry without government permission. Eventually, Mary did marry and recovered her ticket of leave, but until she received certification by a hospital surgeon, she could not legally set up her midwifery practice. Unlike Irving, Mary Mumford was able to successfully navigate through the government bureaucracy to reach a level of social and professional acceptability that afforded her a comfortable working-class life in Maitland as a midwife until her death at the age of 75.

The First Fleet was the first British settlement group, arriving in Australia in January 1788 to establish the penal colony of New South Wales. For most of these settlers, convicts and government personnel, families were left behind in their homelands, and they were now separated from community medical support systems and traditional health practices. The only available orthodox medical treatment was provided by the naval surgeons who accompanied the fleet.

Initially, the colony ran as a quasi-military operation with a social hierarchy unlike that of the colonists' homelands. The social structure was not one where all previous social standards were wiped clean to start a new society based on new standards. Instead, it was a palimpsest built on a melange of social values held by the governor of the colony and his officers, and in varying degrees by the 732 convicts, the 245 marines and the 54 wives and children of marines who made that first journey.[13] These values were the keystone of what was to become the Australian middle-class culture.

Cultural values are the beliefs, principles, and norms to which a society aspires. Among the social building blocks of colonial Australia were evolving conventions that are commonly referred to in archaeological research as middle-class values. In literature and scholarship, the most oft-mentioned of these are cleanliness, sobriety, hard work, chastity and piety. These are collective traits of respectability that meet the real, though vague standard aspired to by the middle class.[14] However, they should more aptly be called "Victorian values", a term used hereafter to identify these conventions that influenced all social classes during not only the Victorian era, but the long 19th century.[15] Research into colonial health repeatedly encounters reference to the role of these values in promoting health and wellbeing.[16] In archaeological scholarship, there is an abundance of research on the influence that class values had on social interaction, but it lacks a discussion on the role these values played in health.

Understanding Australian colonial health in its cultural setting serves to further demonstrate the relationship between Victorian values and their effects on public and personal health during the Victorian era of Australia. These core social values promoted wellbeing in the culture through clean-living habits that improved public and personal health. Furthermore, these values played a notable role in Australia's colonial health, as evidenced in the archaeological record. To achieve this understanding first requires the identification of those Victorian values that can be demonstrated in the archaeological record. Exploring the themes of environmental and social reforms as expressions of these values involves investigating the documentary and archaeological evidence to determine the extent to which they impacted Parramatta residents.

The archaeological record affords opportunities to answer questions regarding class structure, health and approaches to medical treatment. The ultimate goals of this research project are to determine the extent of residents' adherence to or rejection of social conventions and to identify class-related patterns in their attitudes towards

---
12 Salt 1984, 37–9.

13 Gillen 1989, 445.
14 Briggs 2006, xv.
15 Briggs 2006; Young 1988.
16 Beaudry, Cook and Mrozowski 1991; Beaudry and Mrozowski 1988; Fitts 1999; Hayes 2014.

and engagement with these values including potential discrimination in providing health care and environmental health improvement to the lower classes. This requires an assessment of the adverse environmental issues confronting Parramatta settlers during the 19th century, their harmful health effects and how the settlers attempted to alleviate them both through environmental reforms for the collective settlement and individual efforts for private properties.

Numerous detrimental environmental conditions, such as poor drainage and lack of sanitation, affected the settlers' health. In the archaeological record, reforms to address these conditions are best demonstrated by structural remains of government initiatives and private landowner efforts to combat inadequate drainage, public water supply, storm drains and sewerage. Private environmental reforms consisted of dams, drainage systems and sumps that resulted from individuals' efforts to confront issues on their own properties.

Furthermore, examining social reforms that directly and indirectly improved individuals' health through modifying social behaviour contributes to the interpretation of social values. As noted, Victorian values are social conventions that demonstrate respectability (cleanliness, personal hygiene, sobriety, piety, chastity, hard work and honesty). Piety, chastity, honesty and hard work are intangible values primarily recorded in historical documents. Cleanliness, personal hygiene and sobriety leave tangible evidence in the archaeological record that can enhance the historical record. Archaeological evidence of social reforms is best shown by analysing artefact data associated with alcohol and tobacco consumption but with particular attention to the cessation of consumption promoted through temperance reform movements. To a lesser extent, artefact data furthers the understanding of the social values of cleanliness and personal hygiene. Interpretation of archaeological data considers historical and sociocultural documentation to determine the degree of success of these social reforms.

Parramatta in the long 19th century

The chosen timeframe is the "long 19th century" (1788–1900s), encompassing Australia's colonial era and therefore the late Georgian period (1746–1837) and the Victorian period (1837–1901) in the colony. The European colonial community was selected because this was the segment of the population that embraced Victorian values and Parramatta is the setting for my case study.

Parramatta is one of the earliest settlements in New South Wales. It was established as an agricultural outpost in late 1788, only ten months after the initial convict settlement at Sydney Cove when the latter proved to lack arable land. Its riverfront location 25 kilometres upriver from Sydney allowed for ready food supply to the main settlement (Figure 1.1). Parramatta quickly transformed into a free settlement and within a few decades had expanded from a rural outpost to a thriving pastoral centre and market town. A new and loosely grouped class of pastoral businessmen were key players in transforming the convict settlement into a regional agrarian commerce centre. The 1855 arrival of the railway improved transport of commodities such as wheat, wool and livestock. The 1850s New South Wales gold rush not only helped bring Parramatta out of the 1840s recession[17], it created a boon, for as diggers rushed westward towards the goldfields, they passed through Parramatta and for a time elevated its commercial importance above that of Sydney. By the turn of the 20th century, Parramatta was more than a market centre, with its rail and waterway connections transforming it into a main transport centre for industry.[18] This social, economic and civic development pattern makes Parramatta an ideal case study for exploring colonial health.

Urban redevelopment of Parramatta during the 21st century has resulted in numerous large-scale archaeological investigations of 19th-century and early 20th-century sites. These investigations afford us an opportunity to look beyond a single site to identify healthcare patterns for the community at large in different time periods. Part of the process is to establish a method to combine these big urban datasets – generated by different artefact analysts using different protocols – into alignment for a multi-site synthesis. As the author was the original analyst for a number of these projects, this made this task considerably more straightforward.

Almost without exception, commercial heritage consultants have conducted archaeological investigations in Parramatta as part of pre-development legislative compliance studies. Commercial site reports are generally limited to archaeology, zooarchaeology, ethnobotany and history, and make only basic interpretations of the sites' residents' lives. These archaeological studies have identified several public infrastructure initiatives across the Parramatta landscape, such as drains, dams and landscape or environmental modifications. To enable research into the personal health issues of those who lived in Parramatta in the long 19th century, residential sites were selected because they provide the most substantial datasets on people's everyday lives. Eight of these residential sites were chosen based on four criteria: sealed rubbish deposits; long-19th-century date range; a cross-section of social classes; and identified resident(s) associated with the location and deposits. In addition, the site of Parramatta's oldest pharmacy, which operated from 1831 to 1880s, was included for comparison to household self-medication practices.

Medical anthropology

Medical anthropology provides a theoretical framework for historical, sociological and archaeological research, analysis and interpretation. Using a medical anthropology approach enables an understanding of the fundamental

---

17 Dyster 2022.
18 Kass, Liston and McClymont 1996, 260–2.

1 Nineteenth-century health and Victorian values

importance of sociocultural relationships in health and illness. Much like a holistic medical practitioner's approach to treating a patient by respecting the mind, body, spirit, emotions and environment of the patient, medical anthropology integrates biological, cultural and social factors to build a unified theoretical understanding of the origins of ill health in a culture.

The merger of research from several disciplines allows for the development and formulation of research questions and facilitates historical research and archaeological site selection and data synthesis. Part of the framework involves forming a methodology for site selection that incorporates several different theoretical approaches[19] to analyse and interpret artefact collections without the imposition of preconceived patterns. This framework also requires having sufficient sample sizes of alcohol, medicine and hygiene-related artefacts, and that there is historical research that links the collections to a documented household or individual. Beyond the basic site-selection criteria, the chosen sites also had either archaeological evidence of localised environmental reforms, such as drainage infrastructure, or documented geographic assessments explaining the lack of necessity for such reforms. Features and deposits within each site could help answer questions related to both environmental and social reforms.

Social structure is just one component of a culture. But, as Ruth Benedict discussed in *Patterns of culture*, it is not possible to understand one trait of a culture without an understanding of the culture as a whole.[20] Comprehending Parramatta's history, the development of Australia's health systems and the evolution of the colony's social culture are essential building blocks. The colonial culture was not static, and the evolution of social structure is crucial to perceiving the influences Victorian values were able to assert. There were many contributing factors to what became known as the Australian ethos, including the self-improvement attitudes of radical "gold-rush" immigrants, the conservatism of the pastoralists, the influence of the clergy through their magisterial role in the colony, and resentment of the middle class by the working class. The middle class was a part of the social structure from the time of the First Fleet. By the 1830s, the middle class was not emergent but rather had insinuated itself securely between the working class and social elites, including the pastoralists (often deemed the Australian aristocrat group). As overseers of the working class, they pressured the workers to conform to generally held social values. This pressure was imposed as a form of control and a campaign to improve the morals and manners of the working class.

The research outlined in this book uses archaeological analysis of environmental and social reforms in Parramatta to demonstrate the extent to which Victorian values influenced the health of Parramatta's residents through studies of infrastructure and artefacts. It demonstrates the level of influence these values asserted over colonial society, particularly the health of the Parramatta community. Furthermore, the analysis shows the development of the emerging Australian culture, its role in improving available health care and its effects on Parramatta's population. While these results speak only to conditions in Parramatta, they represent a model for comparative studies on this topic in other Australian regions and urban settings during the colonial era.

Organisation of this volume

Medical anthropology is the foundation for this book's discussion of historical, health and sociological research that is then used to interpret archaeological research for a city-wide case study for 19th-century Parramatta. A prerequisite to the case study is an overview of Parramatta's history as it relates to health and sociocultural development, told through the lives of Parramatta's residents, its medical practitioners and prominent personalities (Chapter 2). The city-wide case study developed for Parramatta incorporates the basic site-selection criteria of artefact collections with sufficient sample sizes from sites with documented households or individuals and archaeological evidence of localised environmental reforms that could address questions related to both environmental and social reforms (Chapter 3). Chapter 4 argues that an understanding of the evolution of social structure resulting from social reforms is crucial to determining the influences Victorian values could assert on the health of Parramatta's residences. The discussion of Victorian values and their health implications in Chapter 5 requires their recognition as markers of respectability while acknowledging that they served to promote good health within the community. A review of relevant medical history (Chapter 6) is a prerequisite to discussing public and private health and presents a background of health conditions in the early colony. A discussion of public health and environmental reforms to improve public health, including historical and archaeological evidence, demonstrates the extent to which Victorian values influenced Parramatta's residents' health through studies of infrastructure improvements (Chapter 7). In Chapter 8, the archaeology of personal health examines how social reforms promoted wellbeing through proactive and reactive health care and how healthy lifestyle patterns, or the lack thereof, are demonstrated in the archaeological record.

The overarching theme that connects all chapters is an examination of historical, archaeological, medical and sociological evidence within the framework of medical anthropology to examine social conventions and their influence on health in 19th-century Parramatta. The research addresses basic inquiries designed to examine the evidence to clarify cultural values' impact on cleanliness and health. The discussion in Chapter 8 is designed to answer the question: Did Victorian values dominate approaches to health in the colonial social system?

---

19 Agency, structuration and post-processual theories.
20 Benedict 1934.

Chapter 2
BRIEF HISTORY OF PARRAMATTA

Before the first colonial settlers came to the area, the Burramattagal of the Wangal clan had lived on this land for 60,000 years. These traditional owners lived in groups of 30 to 60 people, following seasonal routes within territorial boundaries.[1] The Burramattagal people were attracted to the area for the abundance of eels, fresh fish, crayfish and turtles the river's fresh waters provided, and they referred to this area as *parramatta* ("many eels"). Food gathering on land included trapping and hunting animals and gathering insects, their eggs and larvae. Plant foods were also abundant, with berries, plant seeds and fruits readily available for gathering.

Within months of the arrival of the First Fleet in January 1788, the colony's survival became precarious. Inadequate soil conditions for agriculture in the Sydney Cove area necessitated the search for more arable land elsewhere. An area later called the Crescent was identified upriver from Sydney on the Parramatta River. Here, the rich silt deposits created by the weathering and erosion of igneous outcroppings upstream had been deposited, creating fertile areas for the cultivation of crops.[2] Rose Hill, later renamed Parramatta, was the settlement established in November 1788 adjacent to the Crescent to accommodate the convicts and overseers who farmed the crops to feed the colony. The first settlers in Parramatta were seven officers, 20 marines and 20 convicts, who were sent out to clear the site and construct rudimentary structures.

As a result of successful crops, the Parramatta settlement thrived, and soon free settlers (mostly decommissioned officers and marines) began to take up agricultural and pastoral land grants in the surrounding countryside. Its colonial history can be chronicled by a timeline of events set in a series of time periods that represent the stages of the town's evolution (Table 2.1). Firsthand observations provide details that further our understanding of the evolving physical, geographic, socio-economic, religious and stewardship environments that influenced their lives,[3] while the *Historical Records of New South Wales* contain government reports and correspondence with details pertinent to regulations and initiatives that were key to the establishment and development of Parramatta.

Woven into the chronicles of Parramatta's history are accounts of the people who settled and developed the town. But also woven into this history are the records of its health care and social development structure and how changes in these systems affected the lives and health of its residents.

Time period 1 – convict settlement (1789–1820s)

For the earliest Europeans, the struggle for survival and wellbeing can be seen through the lives of two men: farm supervisor Henry Dodd and surgeon John Irving. The rush to produce sustainable crops was exacerbated by an inadequate administration that failed to include a farmer to oversee and manage agricultural activities.[4] After initial difficulties, the supervision of the Parramatta farm was left to Henry Dodd.

Henry Dodd was a farm labourer who had worked at Lyndhurst in England for Arthur Phillip, the colony's first governor. He was given a chance to start a new life in a new land. Whatever Phillip's original intention, by March 1790 Dodd found himself the second superintendent of convicts employed in cultivation at Parramatta.[5] Dodd's success as farm supervisor was due more to his ability to oversee convicts without military coercion than his farming skills.[6] By 1790 Dodd reported that there were 200 acres[7] of cleared and cultivated land, including an estimated 55 acres of wheat and barley that would yield 400 bushels.[8] This quantity of grain would produce 24,000 pounds of wholemeal flour when equipment to grind wheat finally arrived with the Second Fleet in June 1790.[9] Crops were not the only issue Dodd faced, with one report noting that hogs did not thrive or multiply due to the lack of food. Ignorance of local flora and fauna further limited the colonial diet, and plans to establish a dairy were thwarted when, shortly after landing, the four cows and one bull escaped and were not recovered until 1795.[10]

John Irving was one of 11 surgeons who arrived in the First Fleet and the only convict on a medical team servicing 1,400 convicts, soldiers and administrative staff. A certified surgeon, Irving had his skills first noted by the surgical superintendent on the British prison

---

1 Kass, Liston and McClymont 1996, 3–7.
2 Bennett 1865, 125.
3 K.M. Brown 1937; Hassell 1902; Jervis 1963; Kass, Liston and McClymont 1996; Tench 1793a; b.
4 Kass, Liston and McClymont 1996, 17.
5 Kass, Liston and McClymont 1996, 17.
6 Collins 1798, 101.
7 One acre equals 0.404686 hectares.
8 Tench 1793b, 55.
9 Clements 1986, 32.
10 Clements 1986, 32.

Cleanliness is next to godliness

Table 2.1 A Timeline of key events in Parramatta's history. Source: Parramatta Heritage Centre 2015.

Time period	Date	Event
1. Convict settlement (1789–1820s)	18–20 January 1788	First Fleet arrives at Botany Bay
	November 1788	Parramatta settlement established
	1789	First crops harvested
	1790	Parramatta Town laid out
	1791	Officially renamed from Rose Hill to Parramatta
	1796	First church opens
	1804	First brewery opens
2. Market town (1820–1830s)	1821	Parramatta Female Factory completed
	1832	King's School opens
	1836	Lennox Bridge built
	1840	Convict transportation ends in New South Wales
3. Moving forward (1840–1860s)	1843	First newspaper (*The Parramatta Chronicle*)
	1860	Railway arrives at Parramatta Station
	1861	Incorporated as a municipality
	1868	Convict transportation ends in all colonies
4. Feast and famine (1870s–1900s)	1873	Gas turned into town mains
	1888	Centennial Baths open
	1890	Friendly Societies form United Friendly Societies' Dispensary and Medical Institute
5. A new nation (1901 onwards)	1910	Sewerage scheme completed

hulks, where he spent the first four years of his seven-year sentence. While there is no record of his surgical services during the First Fleet's voyage to the colony, upon arrival he was immediately employed as an assistant surgeon to Chief Surgeon John White. Irving was then assigned as assistant surgeon at Parramatta Hospital in 1791. His conduct and behaviour were so praised that Irving became the colony's first emancipated (pardoned) convict.[11]

In Parramatta, Irving found a temporary hospital that was not much more than two long thatched-roofed canvas-walled sheds. The second hospital, a permanent structure built in 1792, had a 200-patient capacity but overflowed with nearly 400 patients on any given day.[12] Through shared experience, Irving was all too aware of the deficient health of his fellow transportees. The first few years after the arrival of the First Fleet were brutal. The threat of death from malnutrition was grave, with widespread dysentery and inflammation ailments due to the insufficient and unbalanced diet. Among the few medicines at Irving's disposal were quinine for malaria, digitalis for heart failure, colchicine for gout and opiates for pain.[13] After malnutrition, infectious diseases were his worst enemy. Germ theory would not be proven until the late 19th century, while the necessity of disinfecting wounds and surgical instruments, and the benefits of clean and sanitary conditions in hospital and surgeries, were not yet fully recognised.

By the time Irving arrived in Parramatta in 1791, the initial food crisis of the First Fleet had been weathered, although shortages continued. More lands had already been cleared under Dodd's supervision and grain and crops had been harvested. Much-needed supplies arrived with Second Fleet, but half of the 760 new convicts were barely alive, and their ill health and inability to be productive members of the colony put yet another strain on the colony's resources, including that of the services of surgeons such as Irving.[14]

Both Dodd and Irving were aware that the colony's survival depended upon raising crops that would maintain some level of health among the settlers. The imported stores were basic and had to be augmented by

---

11 D. Richards 1987, 1.
12 Tench 1793a, 246.
13 Due n.d.
14 R. Hughes 1986, 145.

goods manufactured or grown from local resources. For the first five years, the limited colonial diet resulted in rampant scurvy due to the lack of fresh, identifiable local plant foods. Fortunately, colonial surgeons, like John Irving, eventually found two types of edible local berries (species of *Smilax* and *Leptomeria*) that supplemented vinegar and potatoes as foods to treat scurvy cases.[15] Successful crops and proper milling equipment provided colonists with the opportunity to obtain a balanced diet. Nevertheless, a decade later botanist and explorer George Caley noted, "It was not uncommon to see people in a reputable situation to be without vegetables for some months in the years".[16] Undoubtedly, the situation was more severe for people in less than a reputable situation.

Such was the nature of the hard life that faced European settlement during that first decade in Parramatta. What followed was the development of a fledgling colony. With a somewhat stable food supply, shelter and basic health care provided by the government, the colonists' attention turned to establishing social conventions. Some newly arrived free settlers assiduously strove to re-create the social and moral standards of the homeland in this fledgling colony. Reverend Samuel Marsden, who arrived in 1794, was one of two government-recognised clergy members in early New South Wales who eventually assumed the role of religious leader for the Anglican Church in the colony. Following the common practice in England, Marsden also served as a magistrate for the Parramatta region. With his strict code of what he considered acceptable behaviour, Marsden proved to be stringent in his conviction that convicts and settlers conduct themselves morally and civilly, as he interpreted the law. Marsden was of the opinion, shared by many of his middle-class male contemporaries, that specific lifestyle patterns of convicts and working-class free settlers would only lead to criminal behaviour. Foremost of these were excessive drinking and gambling.

According to Marsden's contemporary, Parramatta pastoralist James Macarthur, the scarcity of beer, wine and cider led to a high rate of consumption of spirits.[17] The government wanted an alternative to spirits, but the shortage of grain and the early threat of famine resulted in a ban on brewing. After several successful crop seasons, Governor King commissioned the construction of local breweries and then took measures to establish a vineyard in 1801. He charged Anthony Landrin (Antoine L'Andre) to establish a vineyard in Parramatta, which saw its first vintage in 1804. In the same year, the government brewery at Parramatta was established, producing 6,000 gallons[18] of beer per week.[19]

By the dawn of the 19th century, many convicts had served their sentences and were free to pursue their own way. Better agricultural land was located elsewhere, and with improved roads and the establishment of a regular ferry service to Sydney, Parramatta quickly grew from an agricultural town into a hub for commerce (Figure 2.1). The first land leases in Parramatta were issued in 1809 with a tenure of 14 years.[20] Many free settlers and emancipated convicts acquired land leases in Parramatta, including of the lots that previously accommodated the convict population.[21] Anthony Landrin was able to acquire a leased lot (Site 7, 2 George Street) with an updated former convict weatherboard cottage (Figure 2.2). As Parramatta transitioned from a convict to a free settlement, these convict cottages were significantly modified or replaced.[22] When emancipated convict Samuel Larkin (Site 7, 2 George Street) took over Landrin's lease in 1824, he added a tile-and-brick storage cellar to his property.[23]

Between 1790 and 1821, the population of Parramatta grew from 260 to 4,778, leading to the freshwater supply from the Parramatta River becoming contaminated. Public wells were sunk in 1813 and 1815 to alleviate this problem and the "Town Dam", located near current Marsden Street where freshwater and saltwater meet, was constructed in 1818. As Parramatta's population continued to expand, the absence of a municipal drainage system became another issue, and landowners of properties in low-lying areas struggled to control dampness and run-off.

Time period 2 – Market town (1820–1830s)

By the 1820s, Parramatta had developed from a small frontier town to a prosperous regional agricultural and pastoral centre. Land and property acquisition became one of the primary issues of this era. As convicts obtained their tickets-of-leave, they were permitted to seek employment for their own benefit, marry and acquire property.[24] Their addition to the existing "at-large" population of free settlers meant economic growth. Also, the population increased as additional free settlers and emancipists gravitated to the town (see Table 2.2).

To better manage the convict population, Governor Macquarie decided to remove convicts from the town and housed them in the convict barracks built in Parramatta in 1821. The remaining former convict cottages were available for occupancy by ticket-of-leave convicts and free settlers.[25] By 1823, when the original 14-year leases from 1809 expired, 342 applications were made for new 21-year leases that represented practically all the allotments in Parramatta.[26] A number of these new town leases were obtained by Parramatta's emerging

---

15 Clements 1986, 30; Maxwell-Stewart 2006.
16 Flannery 1999, 191.
17 Sturma 1983, 146.
18 One gallon equals 3.78541 litres.
19 Kass, Liston and McClymont 1996, 62–3.
20 Kass, Liston and McClymont 1996, 113.
21 Casey & Lowe 2006a, ii.
22 Parker 2006, 38.
23 Stocks 2008, 35.
24 Therry 1863, 509.
25 Higginbotham 1991, 12.
26 Kass, Liston and McClymont 1996, 114.

Cleanliness is next to godliness

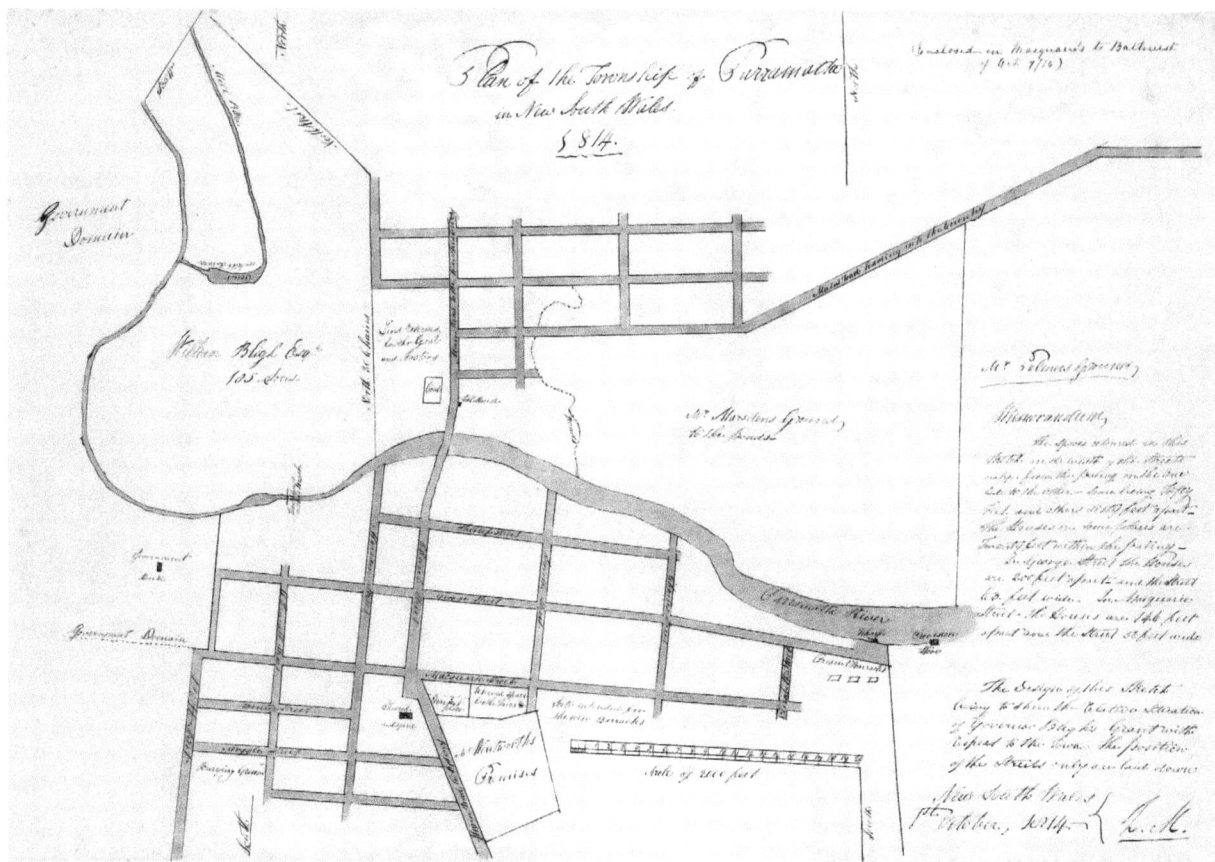

Figure 2.1 An 1814 plan of Parramatta commissioned by Governor Lachlan Macquarie. Source: the collections of the State Library of New South Wales (a1528520/M2 811.1301/1814/1, Mitchell Library).

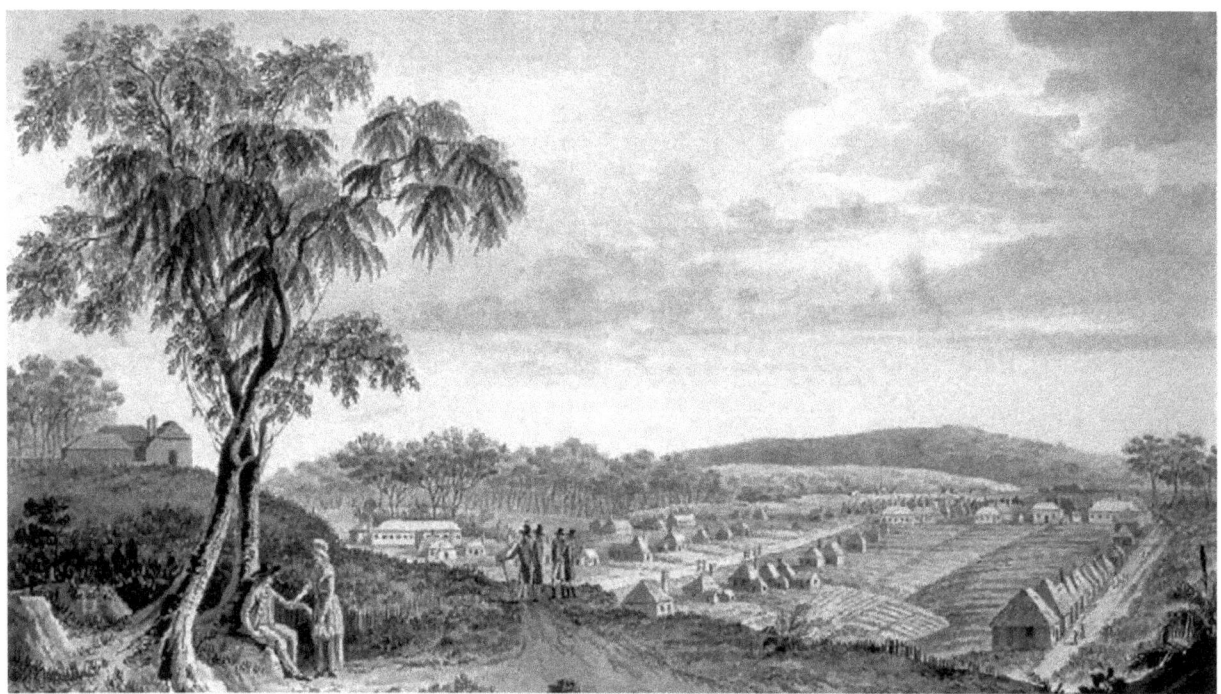

Figure 2.2 Sketch of Parramatta, April 1793, by Fernando Brambila, showing the early convict settlement at Parramatta. Source: Map Library, British Library Board, Maps T.TOP.124 SUPP F44.

2 Brief history of Parramatta

Table 2.2 Parramatta Population Chart 1788–1911. Source: Australian Bureau of Statistics 2014.

Year	Parramatta		Sydney	New South Wales			Australia
	Convict	Total		Convict	Free settlers	Total	
1788						1,480	
1790		260	1,454	1,266		1,714	
1796						2,953	2,953
1801		1,457				4,372	4,372
1804		1,900					
1811						6,675	7,697
1812		2,571					
1821		4,778	12,400	13,814	15,969	29,783	
1828†	1,767	4,618	10,815	15,728	20,870	36,598	44,778
1833†		2,637	16,232				60,794
1836		3,600	19,729	27,831	49,265	77,096	
1841		5,389	29,973			94,094	144,114
1847		4,500					189,609
1851*		4,128	53,924			113,155	256,975
1861*		13,758				201,259	669,373
1871*		11,560				282,150	947,422
1881*						426,933	1,247,059
1891						622,523	1,736,617
1901						720,849	2,004,836
1911						890,578	2,382,232

* In 1882, a fire destroyed the New South Wales census records for 1846, 1851, 1856, 1861, 1871 and 1881, including the detailed household forms from 1861, 1871 and 1881.
† Census year.

gentry, including John Macarthur, Gregory Blaxland, Reverend Samuel Marsden, Dr D'Arcy Wentworth and John Harris. These families also had other large land grants in or around Parramatta or had their Parramatta leases converted to land grants by virtue of substantial improvements they made to the properties.

In Australia, the term "squatter" originally referred to a person illegally grazing his livestock on Crown land, but eventually came to mean a person with a large-scale freehold property (station). Often referred to as the squattocracy, Parramatta's emerging gentry was a loosely grouped class of businessmen, physicians, clergy and government officials who were instrumental in transforming Parramatta the convict settlement into Parramatta the regional agrarian commerce centre.[27] Other leaseholders were middle-class commercial investors like James Byrnes who, through hard work and opportunity, advanced both his social and financial standing. Byrnes had a long career in Parramatta as a contractor and developer with commercial ventures, including a ferry service, a brewery, a flour mill and a textile mill (Figure 2.3).[28]

When Major General Sir Thomas Brisbane arrived in New South Wales in 1821 to be the colony's sixth governor, he chose to settle his family in Parramatta instead of Government House in Sydney because the free settlers in Parramatta included a more respectable class of people among whom his heiress wife and sister-in-law felt socially comfortable.[29] During Brisbane's tenure, much of the colony's formal and informal business was conducted in Parramatta between the governor, wealthy free settlers and long-standing government officials who lived in the area. This interaction served to increase the

---

27 Connell and Irving 1980, 53.

28 Walsh 1969.
29 Kass, Liston and McClymont 1996, 91.

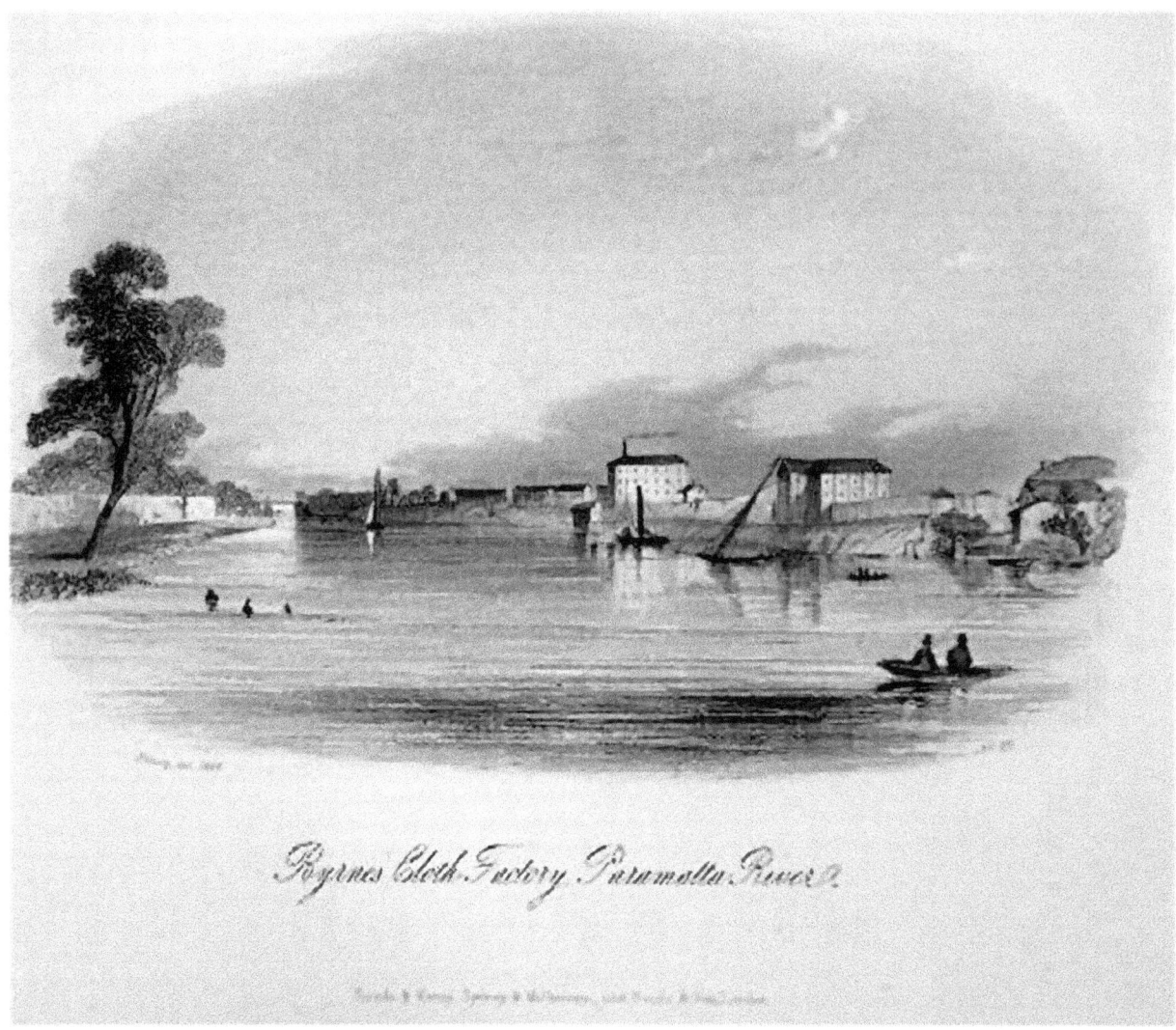

Figure 2.3 Fleury's 1853 view of the Byrnes Cotton Mill located on the Parramatta River. Source: Parramatta Heritage Centre Picture Collection.

town's stature, securing its position as a regional cultural, economic and political centre in the colony.[30]

The town's growth created a need for new and improved infrastructure to address issues of public and private health. A series of barrel drains was constructed in the 1820s to channel stormwater away from low-lying properties, but to some extent, the problem still persisted.[31] For instance, western Macquarie Street and nearby Marsden Street continued to struggle with damp issues that, beyond being a nuisance, affected occupants' health.

Population growth also required improvements to the healthcare system. Parramatta's third hospital, called the Colonial Hospital, was constructed in 1818 and was considered a vast improvement over its two predecessors. Commissioned by Governor Macquarie, the two-storey brick structure included verandahs all round and gardens beyond that afforded patients access to fresh air and sunlight.[32] Macquarie's 1821 removal of convicts to confined barracks also necessitated constructing a separate barracks to house female convicts and their children. Termed the "Female Factory", this institution of confinement included a hospital for the sole use of the inmates, but, by the late 1820s, working-class, underprivileged and destitute women were also accessing the perinatal services it afforded.[33]

The improved health of the colony was evidenced in the wellbeing of the children. During the first few years of colonisation, the mortality rate was high, but common childhood infections were absent until the 1830s.[34] In 1804 Surgeon John Savage, working at Parramatta Hospital, successfully vaccinated children against smallpox for the first time in the colony.[35] Furthermore, the effects of improved nutrition as compared to British

---

30 Kass, Liston and McClymont 1996, 92.
31 Higginbotham 2004, 2.
32 Kass, Liston and McClymont 1996, 87.
33 Salt 1984, 111.
34 M. Lewis 2014.
35 Dyke 2014, S33.

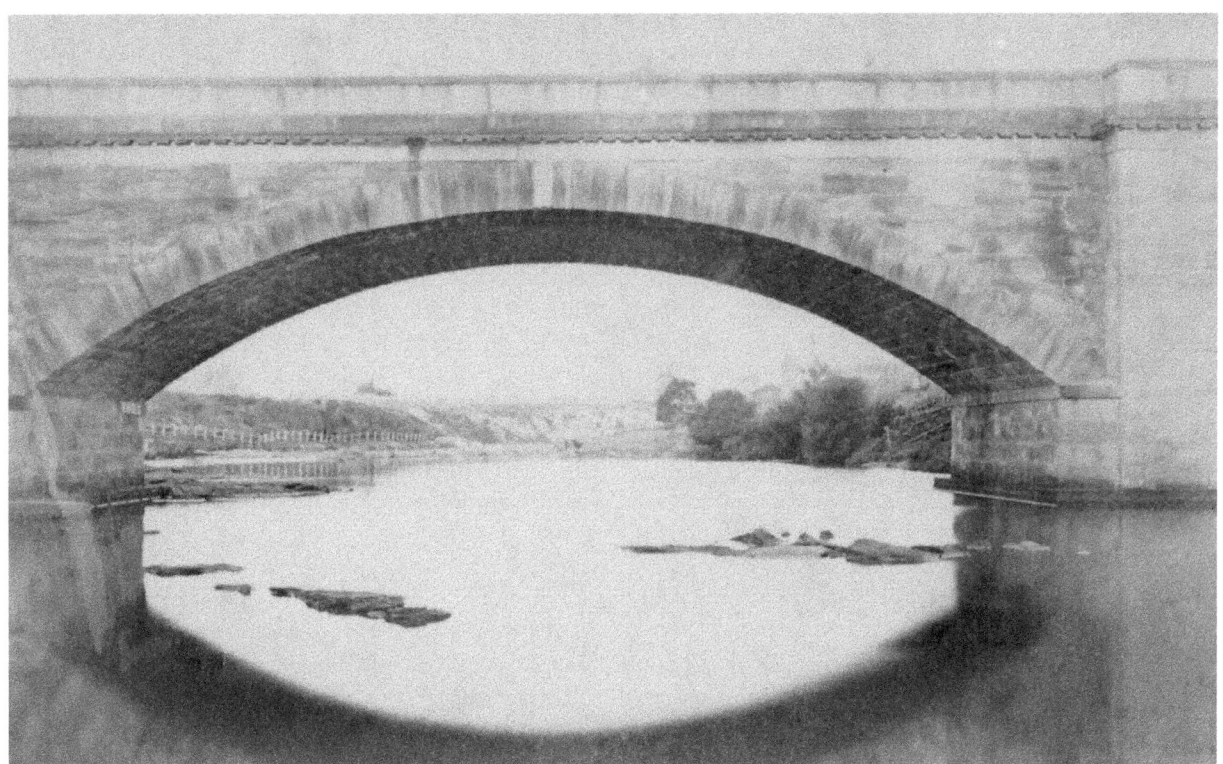

Figure 2.4 The 1839 Lennox Bridge, spanning the Parramatta River, was photographed around July 1870 by Henry Beaufoy Merlin of the American and Australasian Photographic Company. Source: Caroline Simpson Library & Research Collection: 37825.

contemporaries were evident in the increased stature of the first generation of colonial-born Europeans.[36]

The second quarter of the 19th century saw significant medical advancements in developing new pain relief medicines, including morphine (1820s) and codeine (1832). Maintaining personal health became increasingly important during the 1830s, partly due to new and lethal viral contagions sweeping the globe. In 1820 and again in 1825, influenza epidemics hit the colony. A mumps (Rubulavirus, Paramyxoviridae) epidemic struck in 1824 and for the first time in 1828, an epidemic of whooping cough (pertussis) occurred.[37] The government medical services in Parramatta's 1,300–1,600 square kilometre district were stretched so thin that Colonial Surgeon Dr Matthew Anderson could no longer respond to all the calls for his service. The inhabitants of Parramatta took the situation into their own hands and persuaded locally born Dr William Sherwin to set up his medical practice in Parramatta.[38]

Time period 3 – moving forward (1840–1860s)

With the end of convict transportation to New South Wales in 1840, occupancy in the convict barracks gradually dwindled and by 1843 it was converted to a military hospital. Similarly, Female Factory occupancy began to drop below capacity in 1846 but some women were transferred from the asylum, which was overflowing, to the factory and eventually the facility was referred to as the Invalid and Lunatic Asylum.[39] The population of Parramatta had by this time grown eightfold from its beginning to 4,500 persons in 1847 (see Table 2.2).

An economic decline came in the 1840s as the export value of wool was at an all-time low due to the depression in the English textile industry.[40] In Parramatta, a market centre for pastoral and agriculture enterprises, the effects of the depression not only hit successful pastoralists but affected all local tradesmen. The export price of wool and meat dropped to such low levels that tallow for soap and candles was a more valued commodity. As a result, at the depth of the depression, boiling down sheep for tallow became a new and thriving industry in Parramatta.[41]

Until the 1850s, access to and from Parramatta was mostly by water. Within the town, movement across the river had already been improved with the construction of the Lennox Bridge (1836), which was an impressive convict-built structure (Figure 2.4).[42] With the Parramatta Steamboat Company's establishment during the 1840s,

---

36 Maxwell-Stewart 2006, 40–1.
37 M.J. Lewis 2003, 30.
38 *Sydney Gazette and New South Wales Advertiser*, 22 August 1829, 2.
39 Kass, Liston and McClymont 1996, 121; Salt 1984, 121.
40 McMichael 1980, 18.
41 Kass, Liston and McClymont 1996, 134.
42 Kass, Liston and McClymont 1996, 130.

four daily trips were run between Sydney and Parramatta.[43] In 1855, the railway arrived in Parramatta – almost. The line ran from Central Station to Granville at this time, with the remaining 3.8 kilometres to Parramatta's central business district completed in 1860.[44]

By the mid-19th century, two to three generations of Parramatta-born residents were well established in the community, including several who lived at the case-study properties. For example, Hugh Taylor, who was transported with a life sentence in 1815, received his ticket-of-leave in 1821, enabling him to become a constable in Parramatta. By 1824, he had received his absolute pardon. Taylor's son, Hugh Taylor, Jr, attended Parramatta's first private school – the King's School – and went on to be a successful politician and property developer in Parramatta.[45] Australian-born and Parramatta-raised James Byrnes was elected to the first New South Wales Legislative Assembly in January 1858 for Parramatta, just one of many political or governmental positions he held throughout his lifetime.[46]

If one event can be said to be a defining moment in Australian history, it is the 1850s gold rush. Whether a result of the recession, the abundance of available and mobile labourers, or the fever pitch emanating from the California gold rush, the colonial government's decision to open goldfields to prospecting irrevocably changed the shape of the colony.[47] The effects of the gold rush had a positive effect on Parramatta's economy, infrastructure, health care and social structure. Economically, the timing and positive effects of the gold rush on the depressed economy could not have been better. The influx of prospectors saw industries expand to supply basic commodities, such as soap, candles, flour and woollen fabric, for which Parramatta already had a secure place in the market.

Socially, an egalitarian attitude developed in the gold rush, with its belief that "every man deserves a 'fair go'". This new radicalism was the construct of the working class and went against the mid-19th century "image" held by the middle class of their society and social surroundings.[48] This shift would affect cultural development and change the character of Australian culture forever.

Personal health was forgone during the significant influx of gold-rush immigrants who focused more on finding fortune and enjoying the fruits of their labour than ensuring good health. Their diet mainly consisted of mutton and damper, which led to a deficiency of vitamins and minerals, lowering the immune system and rendering a miner more susceptible to colds, fever and disease. Dysentery, fever, scurvy and typhoid were common in the goldfields and often the only treatment sought was that found in a bottle of rum.[49]

Until the late 1830s, the Colonial Medical Service offered free medical care to convicts and free settlers. But, as the population grew and private health care became available, the colonial government gradually shifted to providing medical treatment only for convicts. The transition of management of Parramatta's Convict Hospital (1848) from the colonial government to a local committee of management enabled the facility (renamed Parramatta District Hospital) to minister to all residents.[50] By 1850, there were also ten private physicians.[51] Nevertheless, private health care was expensive and often beyond the financial means of working-class residents. To fill this gap, the Parramatta Benevolent Society, a charitable society that provided social welfare services, used the upper floor of the hospital to tend to female paupers,[52] and working-class friendly societies, such as those in the Loyal Fountain of Friendship in Parramatta (1841), joined together to offer their members medical care at prices they could afford.[53]

Time period 4 – feast and famine (1870s–1900)

As Parramatta's population grew from 8,432 in 1880 to 11,677 in 1890, some original land grants, such as John Macarthur's Elizabeth Farm, Rowland Hassall's George Street estate and D'Arcy Wentworth's south Parramatta lands, were subdivided, sold and developed.[54] In the 1870s, property developer George Coates built a row of semidetached cottages along Smith Street, which are included in this case study. Coates' development was within the southern boundary of Parramatta on the newly subdivided Wentworth Estate, but other developments also sprang up in newly established satellite communities such as Harris Park and Granville. The speculative boom in the property market collapsed in the 1890s and ultimately led to the collapse of the Australian banking system and a severe depression.[55]

During the prosperous 1870s, Parramatta's public utilities expanded to include gas street lighting along George Street, thanks to the creation of the Parramatta Gas Company. Yet the town still had no piped-in water supply.[56] While only three physicians were in private practice in Parramatta in the late 19th century, new medical facilities became available.[57] The Parramatta District Hospital opened a dispensary in 1884, and in 1890 the friendly societies of Parramatta came together to

---

43 Jervis 1963, 59–61.
44 Jervis 1963, 61.
45 Sahni 2016.
46 Walsh 1969.
47 Blainey 1963, 12.
48 C. Taylor 2004, 23.

49 Hagger 1979, 98–9.
50 Kass, Liston and McClymont 1996, 138.
51 Brown 1937, 127.
52 Kass, Liston and McClymont 1996, 138.
53 Jervis 1963, 127.
54 Kass, Liston and McClymont 1996, 213.
55 Fisher and Kent 1999, 22.
56 Jervis 1963, 162.
57 Brown 1937, 123.

form the United Friendly Societies' Medical Dispensary, a clinic to serve its members.[58]

Concern for the colony's public and personal health increased by the last quarter of the 19th century with several new epidemics. Epidemics of scarlet fever and measles in the 1870s caused the worst death rate experienced in the colony (32 per 1,000 people) since those first few turbulent years of European settlement.[59] In 1869 the most publicly debated issue was the proposed compulsory smallpox vaccination. In a letter to the editor in the *Sydney Morning Herald* of Wednesday, 24 February 1869, Parramatta physician Dr George Pringle supported at length the proposed *Infectious Diseases Supervision Act*.[60] Sadly, no such action was taken and the next decade (1880s) witnessed a major smallpox epidemic. Despite these epidemic episodes, the decline in deaths from tuberculosis and other communicable diseases increased the average life expectancy in the late 19th century.[61] At first settlement, the average life expectancy (male and female) was about 35 years, rising to 45 years by the 1870s and almost 60 years by 1900.[62]

By the end of the 19th century, Australia had formed its own cultural identity and there was an agreement among the population that Australia should be self-governed. Sir Henry Parkes spoke best to the dream of Australians in forming their own federation: "We wanted to make these lands the cradle of a more enlightened and more robust freedom than our fathers ever knew. We wanted to build up a fabric of human liberty and human happiness of which they might well feel the utmost pride".[63]

Initially, the consensus in Parramatta was that it was too soon, with many unanswered questions, such as "national defence, the introduction of inferior races into the colonies, and equitable taxation for governmental purposes".[64] By 1898 the questions were focused on the rights of the individual colonies in this proposed federation, and which colonies should be included – implying that the smaller colonies of Tasmania, South Australia and Western Australia should be omitted.[65] Ultimately, Parramatta did not support the 1898 or 1899 referendums for Australian federation. Nonetheless, the Commonwealth of Australia came into being in 1901.[66]

Time period 5 – a new nation (1901)

The dawn of the 20th century saw the end of the colonial era and Queen Victoria's passing. By now, Parramatta had established itself as more than a market centre for the many orchards and market gardens that surrounded it.[67]

With new rail and waterway connections, Parramatta was also the transport centre for industries that had relocated to the nearby suburbs of Clyde and Granville.[68] Noxious industries, such as the Byrnes brothers' boiling-down works (for tallow), slaughterhouses and flour mills were finally shut down or relocated to less populated suburbs, such as Homebush.[69]

The new century brought many medical advancements to New South Wales and Parramatta. New legislation, the *Medical Practitioners (Amendment) Act 1900* (No. 33, 1900), was enacted to impose penalties on people using titles including surgeon or physician if they were not appropriately registered. By 1900, eight Parramatta certified physicians were in private practice.[70] One Parramatta physician, Reginald Bowman, installed one of the newly developed X-ray machines to assist in his diagnoses in his private practice.[71] Also, in 1900, two new wards and an infectious disease ward were completed at the Parramatta District Hospital.[72] The Parramatta United Friendly Societies' Medical Dispensary continued to serve its members until the 1930s.[73]

Long-awaited public utilities and services finally arrived in Parramatta in the 1910s. Water supply was connected to most Parramatta homes and businesses by 1907, and the 50-year wait for municipal sewerage ended with the 1910 completion of Parramatta's sewerage scheme.[74] Electrical lighting replaced gas lighting, and, by 1915, electric power was available to every residence and all street lights were powered by electricity.[75] The original telephone exchange (1893) had had only 16 subscribers.[76] By 1901 that number had risen to 184.[77]

By 1901, the primitive huts of those first convict colonists and their supervisors were long forgotten and unlamented in the bustling town with its modern conveniences.

By the turn of the 20th century, Parramatta residents had time to engage in a variety of leisure activities. Music figured prominently in the community with the formation of several music societies that performed in neighbourhood halls and the acoustically balanced Parramatta Town Hall, and other leisure facilities included a skating rink, a cinema and a merry-go-round.[78] The improved railway service afforded middle-class and working-class residents opportunities to escape suburbia on excursions with clubs and church groups to pleasure grounds and popular seaside destinations, such as Como and Bondi for picnics, and exploration and tramping in bushland.[79]

---

58 Parramatta et al. 2015; Wharton 1911, 124–5.
59 Cannon 1975, 128–9.
60 *Sydney Morning Herald* 19 November 1869, 3.
61 M. Lewis 2014, S6.
62 de Looper 2014, iv.
63 *Sydney Morning Herald* 2 May 1894, 6.
64 *Evening News* 3 May 1894, 3.
65 *Cumberland Argus and Fruitgrowers Advocate* 7 May 1898, 11.
66 Kass, Liston and McClymont 1996, 247.
67 Jervis 1963, 198.
68 Kass, Liston and McClymont 1996, 260–2.
69 Kass, Liston and McClymont 1996, 266.
70 Sands Directory 1900, 1256–9.
71 Brown 1937, 124–5.
72 Parramatta Heritage Centre 2015.
73 Sands 1931, 720.
74 Aird 1961,161–3.
75 Kass, Liston and McClymont 1996, 283.
76 Jervis 1963, 158.
77 A.H. Freeman n.d., 67.
78 Kass, Liston and McClymont 1996, 289–90.
79 Forbes 2016, 8.

Chapter 3
CREATING A CASE STUDY

The Parramatta case study was developed to investigate themes pertaining to the influences of social values for good health in New South Wales during its colonial era. It includes data from a series of sites representing a cross-section of Parramatta's social structure, selected from more than 100 archaeological consultancy reports. These heritage consultancies, undertaken with government oversight to ensure consistency in the recording and reporting, present a high level of documentation of field and laboratory processes and provide a body of data with untapped research potential. The criteria for site selection enabled a line of inquiry based on results generated from archaeological collections (both structural remains and artefact data). While site-specific research topics have been the subject of journal articles and paper presentations, there are no large-scale comprehensive or city-wide studies on Parramatta that utilise this extensive resource.[1] When a city-wide perspective is taken, it is possible to identify patterns of cleanliness for health-related issues in a progression of 19th-century time periods and within different social classes.

Case study: city-wide Parramatta

The intent of this study was to expand understanding of the influences of Victorian values on health and cleanliness beyond the usual focus on a single household by employing a city-wide perspective. This approach interprets archaeological data from multiple sites to determine how social values affect health in a community. This method is not novel, but one that has been employed in numerous earlier studies. One of the first works to use a city's archaeological landscape as a single urban site was Cressey and Stephens' 1977 city-wide archaeological plan for the Alexandria, Virginia, Urban Archaeology Program.[2] City-wide archaeological plans set out standards for systematic and consistent data collection from archaeological investigations, and the city of Alexandria was one of the first to address urban settings in America. In 1981, the Charleston Museum in South Carolina produced a city-wide research plan that enabled Zierden and Reitz to systematically synthesise faunal data from archaeological investigations spanning nearly 50 years.[3]

Similar archaeological management plans have been produced for cities throughout Australia.[4] Parramatta's 1989 Archaeological Zoning Plan (AZP) was the first broad-scale archaeological zoning plan undertaken in Australia.[5] Taking up where the AZP left off, the 2000 Parramatta Historical Archaeological Landscape Management Study (PHALMS) was one of the most detailed and ambitious urban archaeological management plans in Australia for its time.[6] It was a regional study that attempted to identify every parcel of land and every past or existing built structure, producing a framework for a standardised assessment of properties representing Parramatta's rich 200-year history of European settlement. PHALMS consisted of an expanded study area and strengthened thematic structure. Furthermore, it recognised a lack of synthesised publications on Parramatta archaeology that might contribute to the archaeological resource on a state, national or global level. PHALMS also provided the framework for a systematic synthesis of data for Parramatta sites used in this study.

Urban redevelopment of Parramatta during the 21st century has resulted in several large-scale archaeological investigations of 19th-century sites that present an opportunity to look beyond a single site to identify patterns in health concerns for the community at large.

Archaeological site selection criteria

Health-related themes in this case study are analysed by examining both recorded archaeological features (drainage systems and water supply) and data for artefact assemblages that allow us to identify the health issues facing Parramatta's 19th-century residents. Eight residential archaeological sites were selected for inclusion in the case study. Additionally, more than 30 heritage consultancy reports, articles, books and plans contributed historical and archaeological information for background and comparative purposes.[7] Of note are Parramatta archaeological resources outside the case study that had identified archaeological features that furthered the understanding of Parramatta's drainage issues, including evidence of the government's public health initiatives[8] and those initiatives on private property that served to

---

1 Harris 2021, 29.
2 Cressey and Stephens 1982, 41–62.
3 Zierden and Reitz 2016.

4 Iacono 2002.
5 Higginbotham and Johnson 1989.
6 Godden Mackay Logan 2000.
7 Harris 2021, 185–6.
8 Dusting 2016; Higginbotham 1981.

illustrate the extent of drainage issues.[9] Furthermore, artefact collections from archaeological investigations on commercial sites were included as comparative studies: inn and hotel collections in Parramatta were used for comparative analysis on public drinking patterns,[10] while the artefact collection from Parramatta's only documented 19th-century chemist shop was used in a comparison of available patent medicines in a self-medication study.[11]

Residential sites provide the most substantial archaeological data on the everyday lives of the people. The first aspect of data synthesis looks for evidence of individual property owners' attempts to deal with the issues that arose in the absence of government public health initiatives (water supply, drainage and sewerage) – issues that affected their health and wellbeing. The second aspect looks at artefact collections for evidence of health concerns, specifically through analysis of alcohol bottles, medicine containers, personal hygiene items and tobacco pipes.

Eight residential archaeological sites were selected for inclusion in the case study based on the following criteria:

- The archaeological site had a residential use.
- Sites possessed features that demonstrate efforts to control drainage, or in the absence of such features, an assessment of the site's geographic location establishes why drainage measures were not necessary.
- Selected from the archaeological record were structural features (cisterns, privies, wells and cellars) used as rubbish disposal receptacles after abandonment.
- Analysis of the artefactual content of each abandoned feature produced a concise date range for the material.
- Historical documentation was available for the occupants of a site for the time period associated with the selected feature or features.
- Selected sites, features and occupancy are representative of different decades of the long 19th century.
- Sufficient documentation is available to assess each resident's social class and socio-economic status associated with the selected abandoned-feature deposits that meet the above criteria.

For sites that met the criteria, a review of archaeological reports was conducted to identify archaeological features with the potential to supply sufficient data relating to both environmental and social reforms. While the interpretation can be biased by the suppositions of the investigator, each report was prepared with consideration of PHALMS, following guidelines set forth by the New South Wales Office of Environment and Heritage and with a research design that was reviewed and approved by its staff. This government oversight ensured analytical consistency across the body of data generated for Parramatta's archaeological record.

Using structural and geological evidence from across Parramatta enabled the identification of public health initiatives and case studies of residential sites to identify the environmental impact of poor drainage and inadequate water supply to individual homes. Sites were selected based on their ability to meet the research design.

As post-processual archaeological theories demonstrate, there is no fixed, true or definitive interpretation of an archaeological site; the suppositions of the present bias any interpretation of the past.[12] While the data generated from archaeological investigations might represent "hard science", the interpreter's perspective influences the interpretation of that data. This means that, while the findings presented in this book are accurate/true as far as the investigator can make them, they may inevitably be seen differently by other investigators, now or in the future.

Environmental reforms: public and private health initiatives evidenced in structural remains

For the first several decades of colonial New South Wales' existence, occupational and environmental health received little thought. Economic and technological advancements were achieved at the expense of community and workers' health. Increased urbanisation and industrialisation in the growing colony brought increases in environmental and occupational hazards. Newspaper archives contain numerous open letters calling for sanitation reform in Parramatta.[13] Ultimately, the onus was on the government to improve the public health of its citizens. The time had arrived when the need for public health initiatives outweighed the infringement on the individual's personal rights. For example, evidence of this can be seen in archaeologically uncovered remnants of a barrel drain constructed to channel excess water into nearby waterways.[14]

A re-evaluation of archaeological investigations is included here to identify features that evidence attempts to solve drainage issues on private property. The historical record and archaeological site investigations contribute to our knowledge of public environmental reforms. In the archaeological record, structural features – such as wastewater pipes and abandoned cisterns, privies and wells – are evidence for installing municipal services. The historical records regarding the installation of services to individual addresses are sparse for Parramatta and accounts such as Aird's 1961 volume *The water supply, sewerage and drainage of Sydney* are limited to dates for the starting and completion of such public health initiatives.[15]

---

9 Kottaras 2009.
10 Harris 2005; 2019.
11 Carney 1996.
12 Johnson 2010; Shanks 2007.
13 Harris 2021, 187–8.
14 Higginbotham 1981; 1983, 35.
15 Aird 1961.

3 Creating a case study

Social reforms: evidence of personal health practices in artefact collections

Sealed deposits such as wells, cisterns and cesspits are important in this study because they serve as a time capsule for the artefacts they enclose. Analysis of artefactual data requires a methodological framework for artefacts recovered from sealed deposits. A review of archaeological resources found that cesspits as rubbish receptacles have been the subject of numerous articles, including a dedicated volume of the *Historical Archaeology* journal.[16] More recently, an article on the analysis of Sydney's Rocks neighbourhood details methods of assessing cesspit deposits.[17] Wheeler's "Theoretical and methodological considerations for excavating privies" states Schiffer's (1987) formation processes provide the theoretical framework for cesspit analysis for such studies.[18] While construction, use and abandonment processes are the three main behaviours identified for cesspits, this study is limited to use and abandonment processes.

LeeDecker's 1991 study of disposal processes and behaviours associated with the formation of cesspit deposits identifies the accumulation of cesspit fill from the following[19]:

- direct deposition of human and other waste
- accidental loss of objects
- deliberate placement of artefacts and/or materials to serve as percolation fill
- gradual, long-term accumulation of direct household refuse
- rapid deposition of refuse as part of a major cleaning or even site abandonment
- re-deposition of household refuse originally deposited in yards or shed areas.

Schiffer and LeeDecker's analytical approaches to cesspits also apply to deposits in abandoned wells, cisterns and, to a lesser extent, abandoned cellars. The application of these studies makes it possible to determine the manners of artefact accumulation and how the manner of accumulation lends itself to interpreting the data.

Personal health artefact analysis

Beaudry, Cook and Mrozowski present an argument for the importance of symbolism in the interpretation of material culture being used as the basis for the identification of class relationship patterns.[20] The interpretation of material culture requires a foundation of temporal placement and functionality. Standard typologies were established for the Parramatta assemblage as a prelude to chronological reconstruction.[21] For the purpose of functional classification, artefacts were clustered into groups so that statistical analysis of these clusters provided interpretive data on the site.[22] Working within these parameters, each artefact collection could then be analysed for the socio-economic symbols pertinent to this research.

Temporally placed and functionally classified artefacts represent the base starting point for analysis. It is at this point that use-pattern analysis of data begins. Chronological analysis establishes a date range needed to assign time periods to the sites' assemblages and associate them with the resident or residents who lived there at that time. Functional analysis identifies use patterns and enables the interpretation of associated activities. In this manner, research questions are answered and applied to the themes outlined in the research design. Using historical documentation on the occupants of sites sets up comparative temporal and socio-economic status analyses to identify patterns (similarities and differences) in health concerns practised across time and social class. Applying the theoretical framework to these results facilitates an understanding of the agency of Victorian values, cleanliness and health. Details about the sites analysed in this study are provided in the appendix.

---

16 Wheeler 2000.
17 Crook and Murray 2004.
18 Schiffer 1987; Wheeler 2000, 3.
19 LeeDecker 1991.

20 Beaudry, Cook and Mrozowski 1991.
21 Harris 2021, 33.
22 Harris 2021, 48.

Chapter 4
AUSTRALIAN CLASS AND SOCIAL STRUCTURE

From the beginning of colonisation, Australian class and social structure was an evolution of British standards that adjusted for the mix of penal institutions with the free settlers and later the emancipated convicts. The life of wealthy businessman William Wentworth (1790–1882) exemplifies how this structure evolved. Wentworth was the illegitimate son of Colonial Surgeon D'Arcy Wentworth, a quasi-convict (who accepted a post to Australia in order to avoid possible conviction of highway robbery) and Catherine Crowley, a transported convict. Despite William's being illegitimate and the child of a convict, William's father's social standing in Britain and New South Wales probably contributed to his acceptance by the colony's middle-class society. But William's mistress (later his wife) Sarah Cox was shunned by Sydney society. She was the daughter of two working-class ex-convicts. Sarah's social exclusion suggests that mid-19th-century society was not prepared to overlook her convict heritage or her "promiscuous" behaviour.[1] This exclusion was extended to include her seven daughters, who could not find eligible husbands in the colony; to that end, the Wentworths moved to England for eight years to find husbands for all seven.[2]

The following discussions have a threefold purpose. First, they examine the nature of Victorian values with specific reference to health. Second, they offer a context for Australia's and Parramatta's society and culture. Finally, they provide context and class evidence for the households explored in the case-study sites. By design, this study looks at social reforms through comparative artefact analyses between social classes. A prerequisite to these analyses is the determination of "class" for each resident or family in the case study. Class is an intangible aspect of Australian society whose boundaries are not sharply defined. Class analyst Erik Wright contends that most people understand the concept of class in terms of tangible individual attributes and life conditions, including sex, age, race, religion, intelligence, education, geographical location and so on.[3] To synthesise these attributes requires a brief theoretical understanding of class formation.

Development of colonial class formation

Before we discuss social values and their influence on Australian culture, an understanding of the development of social classes in Australia's past is needed. Class structure is just one component of culture, and, as there is no adequate general explanation for the evolution of complex societies, it is not possible to understand one trait of a culture without an understanding of the culture as a whole.[4] When military personnel set out to govern the colony, they suffered a culture shock that is often experienced when someone finds themselves in a situation where there are aspects of culture that differ from what they are familiar with in their homeland, and to which they knew they could one day return. For most transported convicts, the longing for their homeland, which the Welsh call *hiræth,* was permanent, for they were cut off from any hope of returning to a more familiar landscape. The shattering stress and doubly severe disorientation were more akin to what Toffler refers to as "future shock".[5] It was the constant turmoil of this emerging and changing culture that furthered the sense of uncertainty that persisted into the 19th century.

Many in-depth analyses have been written on the development and character of Australian culture. The most succinct is Richard Rosecrance's explanation that the "founding" of Australian culture was not a solitary act. Instead, it was an evolution that developed over three-quarters of a century, starting with the cultural fragment of British society implanted in Australia in the first half of the 19th century, which retained a remarkable distinctness and fixity and culminated with the egalitarianism of the gold camps.[6] The primary emphasis for cultural development of colonies is the cultural inheritance imported in the process of settlement. In Australia's emergent radical post-industrial culture, Britain was the primary foundational influence.[7]

Australia's early colonial culture was set apart by two components: it was established as an isolated penal settlement, and the Australian ecosystem and geography were unlike any encountered by European settlers before. The resulting development of colonial culture also arose from a series of breaks from the traditions of a British-based, hierarchical value system. The evolving Australian class structure was one such broken tradition.

---

1 Johns 2001, 101.
2 Bogle 1993, 16–17.
3 Wright 2015, 3.
4 Benedict 1934.
5 Toffler 1970, 11.
6 Rosecrance 1964, 275–318.
7 Hartz 1964.

The making of colonial social structure

Australia's colonial class structure had two key demographic groups that were not found in the traditional English class structure: convicts and the pastoral gentry.[8] To comprehend their respective roles in the emerging Australian class structure and the possible archaeological expression of these groups, one must understand the evolution of the colony's social, economic and governmental systems.

Colonial Australia's class structure was far from the egalitarian-held attitudes of modern times. Initially, its character was akin to that of a military penal institution. Under the leadership of a colonial governor and with military supervision for gangs and varied assignments, the convict class structure was a scaled hierarchy based on good conduct, for which convicts could achieve increasing levels of freedom within the colony with a full pardon as the ultimate reward.[9] Changes in this social structure began with the arrival of free settlers several years later. The immigrants arriving in late 18th-century and early 19th-century colonial New South Wales needed the security of a social structure. A hierarchical society was a necessary convention of life for them; as social historian Andrew Hassam explains: "There must be someone to look up to, others to look down on".[10] In the case of the Australian colonial culture, comparison with the parent culture was inevitable. Influences of change on the new colony are demonstrated by how the adjustment of the parent culture achieved the colony's new emerging culture.

A key factor for cultural change was a colonial economic system that was supported by assigned convict labour and an economy based on land. Assigned convicts provided free settlers with cheap labour that furthered the successful establishment of agricultural industries. Convicts were wards of the government, which took action to ensure fair relationships between convicts and the settlers (masters) they served. The establishment of the colony's first *Masters and Servants Act* in 1828 gave convicts the right to report grievances, similar to that afforded to servants in Britain for centuries, instilling convicts with a sense of solidarity that identified them as part of their own social class.[11]

Pastoralists (the "squatters" described in Chapter 2) emerged as quasi-gentry in the Australian class structure. Since the developing colonial classes were based on capital, and land was the principal capital, land grants were a contributing factor in class structure formation. Colonial officers and military or down-on-their-luck British gentry saw immigration to Australia as an opportunity to re-establish themselves. The success of these pastoralists was attributed to several factors: the acquisition of vast tracts of land through grants or leases for agricultural pursuits, convict labour that they needed to develop their properties and, in the absence of landed magistrates, their appointment as magistrates in their districts, overseeing matters that included the supervision and discipline of convicts. From the mid-1820s, wool became a lucrative export to Britain and as flocks increased so did the need for land. Thus, pastoralists constituted the wealthiest men in the New South Wales colony. They were a new socio-economic class not experienced in Britain and are referred to throughout this book as "middle-class gentry".

The second half of the 19th century saw the decline of pastoralists as a political force. This downturn occurred because, while they held economic primacy, they had no lasting political influence.[12] They were politically weak compared to Britain's aristocracy because these colonial rural capitalists were answerable to the British Colonial Office, while the British aristocracy was answerable to the Crown and Parliament. But they held onto their economic advantage, because large pastoral and agricultural landholdings (stations) required only a small labour force, and en masse, New South Wales pastoralists employed more labour than did the government.[13] In contrast, the Australian frontier was not conducive to developing small landholdings, placing any smaller-scale producers at a disadvantage. This dynamic denied many would-be smallholding farmers the opportunity for an independent existence, pushing the workforce into the towns and cities where working-class radicalism abounded. The strength of this rising faction of Australian society further decreased the squatters' political advantage. The economic liberalism of a class that strove to emulate Britain's landed gentry did not withstand the radical transformation that called for greater social and political justice.

The "gold rush" chapter in Australian history added another layer to this ethos. Gold-seeking immigrants, who brought with them an energetic, self-reliant attitude, tripled Australia's population during the 1850s.[14] Their ambitious penchant for self-improvement was imbued with reformism. With their pretence of a quasi-gentry class, pastoralists encountered problems when confronted with Australia's growing working-class liberalism and radicalism. The conservatism of the "squattocracy" was gradually overruled by working-class liberalism, and by the 1890s, the politics of Australian society was distinctively liberal.

Explaining the Victorian middle class is the subject of numerous studies, theses and books.[15] These works frequently detail the middle class within the context of the circumstances and cultures of specific countries, and to describe all such variants is outside the scope of

---

8 Connell and Irving 1980, 51.
9 Gibbs 2012, 78.
10 Hassam 1994, 113.
11 Merritt 1994, 113.

12 Rosecrance 1964, 4098.
13 Shann 1930, 134.
14 Rosecrance 1960, 123.
15 Fitts 1999; Hayes 2014; Terry 2013; Young 1988.

this book. The most pertinent point is that the politics, economy and constituents of the middle class and the values of those constituents varied from country to country and even region to region within some countries. The middle class was defined by more than economic and social conventions. The dawn of the 19th century was a new and exciting chapter in the Western world's history. The industrial revolution, which had started in England during the mid-18th century, was reaching the rest of the world. This change resulted in a gradual shift from predominantly rural agrarian populations to more urban populations. With these changing demographics came increasingly crowded living conditions and new social dynamics. Within the structure of the new urban-based industrial society was the emergence of a new class – the middle class – a new layer of the workforce that blurred the lines between the working class (proletariat) and the aristocracy.

The term "gentility" was initially applied in British society to the lesser classes of aristocracy from the 13th century through most of the 17th century, when it became more broadly attached to people displaying good manners. Gentility is based on control of one's body, oneself in society and oneself in the material world.[16] The rising middle class sought to model itself on these principles, distinguishing itself from the working class below, while aspiring to emulate the aristocracy above. Demonstrating middle-class compliance was not based on wealth, but rather the "fluent participation in a core of beliefs and values".[17]

Australian class structure

Australian society was never a microcosm of Britain, as only a fragment of British society was represented in the first six decades of settlement.[18] A large section of settlers came from the poor houses and unions of the United Kingdom: the convicts, emancipists and expirees were predominant, while settlers from the strong British middle class represented less than half of the Australian population in the years 1829 to 1851. The aristocracy was utterly absent. Thus, during the first half of the 19th century, Australian social classes ranged from the very poor, to working class, to middle class, to middle-class gentry.

Despite the hardships of the first years of settlement, there was no poverty of the kind seen in Britain. Initially, the government was responsible for housing, clothing, feeding and the good health of the colony.[19] When convicts had served their sentences and received their tickets-of-leave, they were free to follow their individual pursuits and were responsible for their own welfare. Generally, these emancipists and convicts whose sentence had expired (ex-convicts) gravitated to the towns and cities where the overcrowding and limited employment opportunities left many struggling for existence.[20]

Emancipists were not the only underprivileged non-Indigenous people in Australia at this time. It is impossible to discuss the disadvantaged without examining the British-assisted emigration schemes. In the 1820s Britain had an overabundance of unemployed working-class labourers. Simultaneously, New South Wales had a perceived need for a larger labour force, and the British-assisted emigration schemes were the solution to both problems. Between the 1830s and 1850s, 195,000 British labourers emigrated to Australia through these schemes.[21] This influx of free settlers gradually flooded the New South Wales employment market and labourers lost power over wage demands, with wages forced down as a result. It also increased the ranks of the impoverished. Most immigrants were from the lowest reaches of the British labour force with many arriving with no money or work prospects.[22]

Another category of impoverished people was that of the free settlers who tried to make a living farming the land. They borrowed capital at exorbitant interest rates to purchase land and stock. When severe droughts came, crops failed and livestock perished, with debtors losing their land to their creditors.[23] Frequently, the families were left destitute and forced to live in hovels, joining the ranks of the poor. Governor King slighted these settlers as "useless to themselves and a burden to the public".[24]

The working class consisted of free settlers, emancipists and convicts, but much more is known about convicts even though they constituted only a tenth of the population during the entire convict era (1788–1868).[25] The working class was generally characterised as manual labourers, with skilled craftsmen such as wheelwrights and brick masters on the fringe between working and middle class.[26] The transported convicts and free settlers who comprised the working class came, most with an intense hatred for the upper classes – in Australia represented by the middle class – and the working class had a philosophical attitude that leaned towards leisure as a primary goal in their existence.[27] The attitudes of "officials" of the early colony towards the lower classes were that they should work hard and keep quiet. This static view of social order did not sit well in the emerging colonial ethos.

There is substantial debate among labour historians about the character of the colonial labour force, particularly convict labourers. Mid-20th-century researchers portray convicts as either a homogenous group with class solidarity

---

16 Young 1988, 15.
17 Young 1988, 15.
18 Rosecrance 1964, 4089.
19 Mann 1979, 45.
20 Rosecrance 1964, 4079.
21 Garton 1990, 23.
22 Legislative Council New South Wales 1835, 304.
23 Garton 1990, 28.
24 *Historical Records of Australia* Series 1, volume 3, 421–3.
25 Richards 1993, 255.
26 Young 1988, 58.
27 Rosecrance 1964, 4188.

or as "a lumpenproletariat imbued with petit-bourgeois values, their resistance widespread but quintessentially apolitical and their class consciousness undermined by internal divisions and acquisitiveness".[28] Either way, convicts and most emancipists had limited social mobility, although there were many instances in which emancipists achieved advancement. While the Australian myth of "a fair go" was true for free working-class settlers, ex-convicts were subject to varying levels of discrimination depending on their trade, finances, and social or family connections.[29]

One study of colonial felonry identifies social divisions as perceived by convicts and by free settlers. At the upper reaches of the convict social hierarchy were the "gentleman" convicts who had special skills (such as literacy) or British-based social status that quickly earned them pardons and appointments to government positions of responsibility.[30] Other social divisions among convicts were imposed by government structure. With the establishment of Parramatta's Female Factory, Governor Macquarie imposed a classification system to segregate the recidivist inmates (crime class) from first-time offenders (other class), with more privileges given to the latter. They had a greater clothing allowance, including a Sunday outfit; a better diet; they could work part-time for personal profit; and they could marry.[31] These privileges could be revoked if the inmate was found to be disrespectful, disorderly or dirty.[32] In 1826, a "middle-class" category was added, which was comprised mostly of pregnant women and nursing mothers.[33]

Assigned convicts of lower-class origins tended to remain within the restraints of the convict system throughout their tenure of sentence and did not advance their position within the system. By 1837, 40 per cent of the New South Wales population were emancipists, but despite the efforts of Governor Macquarie, and ten years later, Governor Bourke, positive assimilation of ex-convicts did not happen for those below the social rank of "gentleman" convict.[34] Even if emancipated convicts successfully assimilated into the population, they were socially caught in limbo between the working and middle classes. Mary Reibey (1777–1855) was one of New South Wales' most successful and prosperous emancipists. She was a hotelkeeper, owner of seven farms and a sealing business in the Bass Strait, but Reibey is probably best known for being a Bank of New South Wales founder. Yet Reibey, like many ex-convicts, was shunned by Sydney society. This slight resulted from the ex-convicts' lack of social graces and knowledge of the middle class' etiquette.[35] Unfortunately, Reibey's rejection by middle-class society is indicative of how many female ex-convicts were treated.

While a considerable amount of scholarship has been written on the British middle class, Australian historiography emphasises the principle that Victorian-era Australians differed from their Anglo forebears. For centuries British class structure was static and mobility between classes was rare: an individual belonged to the class they were born with little hope for change in an upward fashion. Australian perception of class structure was based more on the social philosophy that all men are as good as each other if given a "fair go". However, the conception Australians held of their society and social surroundings was not necessarily the reality.[36] The norm in social imagery is most often the ideal in society. The Victorian middle-class concept was that everyone strove to maintain Victorian values when, in reality, the dominant working class was more radical.

A major aspect of genteel living was the underlying division or separation of gender roles. Men worked in the world and women's domain was in the home. While publicly, men were the heads of their households, responsible for making major family decisions, privately, women were responsible for the household's economy, including the supervision of servants and children. Australian husbands and fathers during the Victorian era did not achieve the same status as their English counterparts. The paucity of adult females in Victorian Australia gave women leverage in their choice of husbands and married women maintained greater independence than their English counterparts, although the Australian father maintained the time-honoured head of household role, preserving the sense of traditional family structure.

In the colonial setting, pastoralists began to resemble the English gentry.[37] Much that is written of pastoralists in the historical record relates to their economic and political position in the colony. Their social class was ambiguous. Pastoralists were considered sojourners because, to these affluent settlers, the colony was but a means to acquire wealth, and once this goal was achieved they might return to their homeland. With this sense of impermanence, they lacked commitment to the colony and failed to exert cultural and social influences that contributed to the Australian ethos.

---

28 Roberts 2011, 39.
29 Cannon 1971, 16–23.
30 Blair 1983, 3.
31 Salt 1984, 80–1.
32 Salt 1984, 70.
33 Department of Environment and Energy n.d.
34 Cannon 1971, 18.
35 Karskens 2010, 333–4.

36 C. Taylor 2004, 23.
37 Connell and Irving 1980, 35.

Victorian values and their health implications

... the early 19th-century middle class created itself by living the life of the middle class.[38]

In 19th-century New South Wales, all social classes were influenced by values stressing respectability. Respectability had no firm definition, but each social class (gentry, middle class, working class and the poor) had a different interpretation of its social conventions. Therefore, as described earlier, the term *Victorian values*, rather than *middle-class values,* is more applicable for addressing the influences and impact of these values. As noted, generally grouped under the umbrella of "respectability" are all associated social conventions, with the most commonly noted characteristics of a respectable person being sobriety, piety, chastity, good personal hygiene and honesty. Bruce Haley argues convincingly in *The healthy body and Victorian culture* that the Victorian middle class was concerned with health over almost, if not all, other issues.[39]

A core premise embedded in Victorian social values was constraint; these constraints not only strove to improve the unhealthy habits of the middle and working classes through the pursuit of cleaner lifestyle habits but also strove to improve the public health issues that affected the community at large. Several of these values merit discussion to examine them as a model for good individual health.

Cleanliness

In 18th-century English society, cleanliness was a cardinal virtue of respectability.[40] The paradigm of cleanliness in Anglo-European history is a construct involving medical pragmatism, religious virtues and social values, which have been intertwined components of cultures for centuries.[41] Smith's extensive study on cleanliness integrates the philosophies and practices of theologians, philosophers and physicians to demonstrate the connectivity between cleanliness, health, religion and culture.[42] She explains cleanliness as more than hygiene praxes; it includes health systems, religious morals and markers for social acceptability.

From the Middle Ages, English culture associated dirt with disease.[43] The call for improved hygiene became of paramount importance during the plague outbreaks of the 16th and 17th centuries. The medical profession was insistent upon regimes of cleanliness in the street and homes and personal grooming, including skin care and clothing. However, at the same time, the profession called for hygienic moderation in bathing, as they thought it opened the pores, allowing contagion into the body.[44] While noted social theorist Michel Foucault discounts healing through baths as the madness of late-18th-century cultural theories, he overlooks the underlying medical theories upon which they were based.[45] In the late 18th century, the promotion of bathing came from various sources. Research into the antiseptic properties of bathing, introduced into military medicine by John Pringle, was instrumental in the eventual acceptance of bathing as both a preventative and a reactionary measure against diseases. His work was instrumental in campaigns for hygienic reforms in British prisons by activists such as Elizabeth Fry.[46] At the same time, the vitalist healthcare movement, which embraced new medical theories, promoted all types of bathing because, to them, the skin was the most important organ of the body.

Cleanliness was also promoted by the Church of England, whose spiritual doctrines professed that physical cleanliness of the body, clothing and surroundings was symbolic practice for the soul's cleansing. The 18th-century founder of Methodism, John Wesley, noted in a sermon that cleanliness was, first, the mark of politeness; and, secondly, purity of mind.[47] Wesley, known for the axiom "cleanliness is, indeed, next to godliness", was neither the first nor the last religious leader to link physical and spiritual cleanliness. During the 19th century, religious leaders such as Christian Scientist Mary Baker Eddy and Quaker Elizabeth Drinker called for the cleanliness of the body to attain spiritual cleansing.[48] Nevertheless, the connection between 19th-century religious conviction and middle-class reforms for cleanliness was more than theological teachings for healing the soul.

Cleanliness was the single most crucial component of middle-class respectability. The newly emerging middle class understood the medical benefits of cleanliness, sought spiritual salvation through clean living and used cleanliness in social situations as a respectability marker that separated them from the lower classes. "The great unwashed" was a derogatory term that referred to the British lower classes, as they were generally deemed dirty and worth less than the middle and upper classes.[49] This slur on the lower classes may have held true for the industrial workers and residents in British crowded urban environments, but it was not necessarily the case in early colonial New South Wales. In the early settlement period, Parramatta had an abundance of fresh water from the Parramatta River for drinking, washing and bathing. Convicts and the working class bathed

---

38 Young 1988, 14.
39 Haley 1979, 3.
40 Porter 1982, 326.
41 Haley 1979, 3.
42 Smith 2007.
43 Wear 2000, 316.

44 V. Smith 2007, 181.
45 Huneman 2008, 630.
46 Matheuszik 2013, 120.
47 V. Smith 2007, 226.
48 Bushman and Bushman 1988, 1217–18.
49 Bulwer-Lytton 1838, x.

openly along the riverbanks. However, during the next 80 years, waterways became increasingly polluted and contamination escalated to the point that in the 1880s the council installed water mains to pipe water to standpipes in the town, and riverside public baths were constructed.[50]

Along with bathing, clean and presentable clothing portrayed to the public evidence of good personal hygiene practices. The outward appearance of cleanliness through seemingly well-appointed attire was almost as important as bodily cleanliness. There was a common desire of all classes to be well dressed in clean clothes. The well-paid members of the 19th-century working class had expendable cash, and clothing and materials were priority purchases.[51] Even convicts took care to have clean clothing.[52]

Sobriety

There is a substantial body of literature by historians and cultural anthropologists on the social patterns of alcohol consumption in various social settings. Archaeologists have an advantage over other disciplines in that archaeological collections afford the opportunity to "explore alcohol-related themes and the modern processes that have dictated patterns of alcohol production, distribution and use".[53] Despite this, few archaeologists have applied historical and anthropological theories on alcohol use and social reforms. One example of these few is Watson's archaeological study on household alcohol consumption in 19th-century New Zealand, which argues there were numerous social problems linked to alcohol abuse, including spousal and child abuse, bodily injury, suicide and poverty.[54] On this latter point, Elliot's study on working-class consumer choice indicates that spending on alcohol has been grossly exaggerated by historians.[55]

Sobriety has both social and health benefits. More than just ablutions, cleansing the body internally called for temperance of alcohol consumption. As supporters of temperance movements, the colonial government and the medical community all had reasons to promote abstention from alcohol consumption. In New South Wales, the government had economic, civic and social reasons to regulate alcohol consumption. Where regulation of the importation of alcohol was principally an economic issue, reforms for licensing of publicans and public houses were more aligned with social reforms designed to combat the ill effects on morals and industry of the lower classes.[56]

Alcohol played a widely accepted and significant role in Australia's history, established in colonial culture even before the First Fleet landed at Botany Bay in 1788. While rum and wine were part of the on-ship rations for marines, Lord Sydney's settlement plan did not include provisions for alcoholic drinks for convicts, colonists or officials once the fleet arrived in Australia.[57] This decision was a purposeful one and part of the plan for convict reform. This plan quickly dissolved, as shortly after arrival a special issue of rum resulted in a wild night of debauchery. During the early convict era, public houses and hotels catered for every social class and became centres of public social life. Rituals surrounding "mateship", male forms of bonding and solidarity, often included the copious consumption of alcohol.[58]

Numerous factors contribute to the history of Australian alcohol consumption patterns, with most historians marginalising patterns, focusing instead on the regulations for the manufacture, distribution and consumption that played significant roles in drinking habits in the colony.[59] Both Lewis and Allen chronicle government policies designed to regulate colonial alcohol consumption,[60] and Dingle and Lewis present statistics on colonial alcohol consumption.[61] Allen's work on temperance and the regulation of alcohol in New South Wales between 1788 and 1856 best discusses moral reforms planned for the founding of the New South Wales penal colony and the social and economic reasons for their failure.[62]

Regulations governing alcohol consumption and public drunkenness of convicts were largely unenforced in Australia's convict era (1788–1868). The first reason was that drunkenness was considered a sin rather than a criminal offence, and, secondly, arresting a convict for public drunkenness served no purpose as they were already serving a sentence for their crimes (the *Summary Punishment Act* of 1825). Furthermore, there was no local legislation in regards to public drunkenness of free settlers.

Regulations for publicans' licensing began in earnest during Lachlan Macquarie's tenure as New South Wales governor (1810–1821). As part of his aim to improve the morals of the colonists, he set fixed numbers of licensed publicans and eliminated the unlicensed publicans in each district. As Allen notes:

> despite the larger fees *and* fines, retailing liquor remained a rough trade under Macquarie, in large part because the system was poorly policed, and thus, there were few incentives to run a respectable house or even to take out a license.[63]

After Macquarie's regulations, there was a series of New South Wales *Licensed Publicans* Acts that were revised

---

50 Larcombe 1973, 1186.
51 Elliot 1988.
52 *Sydney Gazette and New South Wales Advertiser* 3 March 1825, 3.
53 F.H. Smith 2008, 6.
54 Watson 2018, 34.
55 Elliot 1988, vii.
56 Allen 2013, 111.

57 *Historical Records of New South Wales* 1892, 14–20.
58 Roche et al. 2009.
59 Miller 1995, 165.
60 Allen 2013; Lewis 1992.
61 Dingle 1980; Lewis 1992.
62 Allen 2013.
63 Allen 2013, 113 (original emphasis).

and added to the Macquarie-era laws. Most notable was the 1830 Act that overrode the governor's authority to limit licensed publicans in each district and left the decision for the number of approved applicants to the district magistrates. The results in most districts were the approval of all applications for licences, which in turn led to the highest rate per capita of public houses in the colony since first settlement. Not without coincidence, the 1830s also witnessed the highest per capita consumption of spirits in Australia's history.[64] The 1838 *New South Wales Licensed Victuallers Consolidation Act* was the first of several Acts that instituted far more prescriptive requirements on publicans, such as conditions requiring sleeping rooms and sitting rooms, and that publicans continuously occupy the premises.[65]

The effects of alcohol regulations in Parramatta were somewhat different from those of the rest of the colony for these 20 years (1810–1830), due principally to the efforts of the local magistrate, Reverend Samuel Marsden. As both Christian minister and colonial magistrate, Marsden had to balance his moral values with his judicious duties, but his colleagues suggested that his religious convictions influenced his rulings.[66] From the beginning of his tenure, Marsden had a belief that public drunkenness led to other criminal behaviour, resulting in frequent sentencing for this offence. During the Macquarie era, Marsden made a valiant but unsuccessful attempt to ferret out unlicensed public houses by using hired informants to visit suspected establishments and testify in support of conviction.[67] His suspension from his magisterial position in 1822 due to a dispute with Macquarie's successor, Brisbane, left Parramatta without his stern, moral and judicious guidance.

The early temperance reform movements of the late 18th century had religious affiliations with Quaker, Methodist and Baptist churches.[68] Even though Wesleyan Methodists represented only a small percentage of Parramatta's religious population (6.7 per cent)[69] this ministry had had a strong presence in New South Wales since 1820, when Parramatta's itinerant minister Rowland Hassall began holding services in his barn (Site 8). Contributing to the growing temperance movement, the Wesleyan doctrine had one prohibitive condition for admission to the congregation: "Drunkenness, or the manufacturing, buying, selling or use of intoxicating liquors, unless for mechanical, chemical, or medicinal purposes; or, in any way intentionally and knowingly, aiding others so to do".[70]

The temperance movement was not born in Australia, but during the 19th century it flourished here. The increased popularity of the newly formed movements was instrumental in significantly changing attitudes towards drinking and smoking. In colonial New South Wales, the first reform movements were mostly groups organised through regional and local churches.[71] The ultimate goal of most groups was a virtuous change of individual beliefs towards abstaining from drinking and smoking, but realistically their efforts also encouraged restraint and moderation as stepping stones to this goal. Other, more extreme reform groups sought to eradicate all social sins – drinking, smoking, gambling and obscene literature – from society, which as Dingle demonstrates, were a needed balance to the heavy mateship drinking encouraged in the early colony.[72] Reform efforts promoted through public lectures and publications urged colonial governments to pass laws to regulate the liquor trade and tobacco industry. By the late 19th century, one of its most successful campaigns was the lobbying of colonial governments for local-option policies, whereby residents were given the right to veto licenses in their towns or suburbs. Alliances formed within each colony, resulting in the Sunday closings of hotels in all colonies except Western Australia.[73]

Members of the clergy from other denominations, such as Reverend John Saunders (Baptist), Reverend Ralph Mansfield (Methodist) and the Catholic Dean of Sydney, John McEnroe, were also instrumental in early temperance movement activities. From the 1820s, the clergy of various Christian denominations played active and passive roles in temperance reform. In the mid-19th century, more than half the population of Parramatta belonged to the Church of England (57.5 per cent) but the Church of England (COE) did not readily embrace the call for temperance reform. From the early 1820s, officers of the COE were allowed to participate in temperance activities, but the movement had no official standing and not until the 1860s did the COE make a commitment to support temperance reforms.[74]

The congregation of the Catholic Church was the second largest in Parramatta (26.5 per cent), and during the 1840s and 1850s, the dominant temperance movement in New South Wales was the St Patrick's Total Abstinence Society. Aligned with the Catholic Church, it drew its strength from all levels of the Irish Catholic community who "rejected the stereotype of the drunken criminal Irishman".[75] Much like the Church of England, officers and clergy of the Church of Scotland (6.3 per cent of Parramatta's population) supported temperance reform from the 1820s, but in the 1860s the Presbyterians still showed little interest in supporting the first reform legislation, and sufficient support among church officials was not gained until the early 20th century.[76]

---

64 Dingle 1980, 229–30.
65 Wright 2003, 23.
66 Marsden 2010, 30–1.
67 Allen 2013, 113.
68 Smith 2008, 3.
69 *Government Gazette*, 3 November, 1846, 20.
70 Wesleyan Methodist Connection 1843, 22.

71 Tyrrell 2008, 3.
72 Dingle 1980, 227; Tyrrell 2008, 1.
73 Blocker, Fahey and Tyrrell 2003, 76–7.
74 Shinman 1972, 179–81.
75 Allen 2011, 374.
76 Denny 1988, 225–7.

Influences on 19th-century alcohol consumption go beyond the adverse health effects of alcohol abuse. In Britain, during the early 19th century, a public alarm was raised over beer's adulteration.[77] By the last quarter of the 19th century, the widespread publicity regarding the adulteration of brewed beer became more than just a campaign spearheaded by advocates.[78] In reaction to this growing concern the middle class was more influenced than others, and this showed in the decrease in beer consumption at large. Adulteration was not a significant problem in the colonies' domestic beer production. In 1875, 1,200 samples of colonial beer were tested and, while quality was questionable, the samples did not contain any dangerous ingredients.

The first New South Wales census was conducted in 1828, and from 1829 to 1871 there are sufficient data to show changes in the per capita ratio of Parramatta's publican licences to the population. In 1829 the per capita ratio of licences to population was 1:178. In 1828, there were 15 publican licences issued in Parramatta to service 2,673 residents. In the early 1840s, this ratio rose to 1:125, but in 1871, the ratio dropped to 1:413.[79] In 1841, there were 43 publicans' licences issued in Parramatta to service a population of 5,389: a 1:125 ratio. By 1871, the population had grown to 11,560, but the number of licensed houses in Parramatta had dropped to 28: a 1:413 ratio. Between 1829 and 1841, the number of licensed publicans almost tripled, but the population of Parramatta only doubled. This ratio is consistent with the discretionary authority granted to district magistrates under the 1830 *New South Wales Licensed Publicans Act*. The significant drop in the per capita ratio of licensed publicans by 1871 is probably in response to increased prescriptive regulations.

Piety – the role of religion

Traditionally, the clergy were stewards to the body and soul of their congregation, and as the discussions of cleanliness and sobriety demonstrate, the members of the clergy were proactive in promoting healthy lifestyle through their support of Victorian values. At the dawn of the 19th century, this stewardship was threatened on two fronts. The clergy had to adapt to changing social reforms and to the rise to prominence of science in medicine. In his accounts on the origins of English morality, philosopher Friedrich Nietzsche proposed that Victorians had replaced religion with morality.[80] This new morality, which encompassed Victorian values, demanded compliance with its norms, values and ideals.[81] While many historians contend that the Victorian values developed from a moral reform movement that came out of the emerging religious reforms, such as the ministry of John Wesley, Smith and Haley demonstrate that religion was just one of the major avenues through which social reforms were achieved.[82] The clergy promoted these reforms as a means of maintaining a role of guardianship over the souls of their parishioners.

Historically, Christian demoninations have always proactively promoted and maintained good health. The bible states, "your body is a temple"[83] and the clergy used this to validate their active role as medical advisers to their flocks. This role was threatened when the religious leaders and Christian churches were targeted for exclusion as medical advisors through medical reforms set forth by the Royal College of Physicians in London. The clergy fought to maintain its role as medical advisers to its parishioners by shifting the focus of its advisory role in medicine.

During early settlement of New South Wales, when wellness was critical to survival, the medical officer and his staff of surgeons rose to an elevated position over the Church in matters of health and wellbeing. Consequently, the clergy shifted its focus to an advocacy role for convicts' treatment and wellbeing, but by far the most significant contribution of Christianity to health in the Victorian age was its sponsorship of athleticism. During the mid-19th century, the clergy adopted a proactive approach to instilling good health habits in their congregations by promoting sporting events through organised social outings and sport leagues. Termed "muscular Christianity", this new approach had a sustained impact on how Anglo-Christians viewed the relationship between sport, physical health (fitness) and religion.[84] The basic supposition of Victorian muscular Christianity was that participation in sport could contribute to the development of Christian morality, physical fitness and "manliness", or in other words, "the training of a man's body for the protection of the weak, and the advancement of all righteous causes".[85]

The Church of England directly taught these values in its schools. As a lad, Reverend James Hassall was in the first group of Parramatta boys to attend the King's School, started in 1832 by Reverend Robert Forrest of the Church of England. Part of the curriculum included sport at the nearby Harris' Field recreation grounds where the students engaged in sport such as cricket and games such as leapfrog.[86] Outside an academic setting, the church went further to encourage church-organised sport teams and family social outings to nearby pleasure grounds. These activities were often reported in the newspapers and congregational newsletters and frequently included the names of participants.[87] Evangelical priest Charles

---

77 Accum 1820, 113–62.
78 Polya 2001, 9.
79 *Sydney Herald* 10 May 1841, 2; *Australian Town and Country Journal* 5 August 1871, 24.
80 Rosenthal 2019, 1.
81 Robertson n.d., 3.

82 Dillon 2002, 265–79; Haley 1979; V. Smith 2007.
83 1 Corinthians 6:19.
84 D.W. Brown 1987; Watson, Weir and Friend 2005.
85 T. Hughes 1880, 99.
86 Hassall 1902, 13–18.
87 Forbes 2016, 36–38.

Kingsley postulated that, since bodies are temples of the living God, physical health honours and maintains those temples.[88] Kingsley also viewed private school, community and church sporting activities as one step towards blurring the lines of class distinction.[89] By the 1860s athleticism was well embedded in Australian society, but with only token recognition of the religious element.[90]

Members of the clergy were also instrumental in the social and religious reforms of convicts. In particular, the Anglican clergy (Samuel Marsden excepted) were proactive in the reformation as they were expected to rehabilitate the convict population for the benefit of the church and of society. The Catholic clergy generally held an opposing opinion, feeling that convicts were lost souls with little chance of salvation. Nevertheless, some Catholic clergy supported governmental reform efforts for the treatment of convicts, such as those of Governor Bourke's 1832 *Summary Punishment Act*, which restricted the scope of sentencing by a magistrate while sitting alone on the bench.[91]

Work ethic

For the Victorian middle class, work was a value achieved through self-discipline with benefits to the individual through improved mental and physical wellbeing, as well as contributing to the potential for economic stability and improved social standing. "Early to bed and early to rise, makes a man healthy, wealthy and wise", an oft-quoted maxim from a book by Benjamin Franklin, was taken on as a mantra.[92] The inference was that one would benefit by rising early and engaging hardily in daily work. This adage may have seemed absurd to the working class, as these hard-working men and women were already going to bed early in order to rise early and go to work, often to hard or repetitive labour that destroyed their health and had little economic benefit.

In early colonial society, a "get-by" attitude prevailed among the convict and working classes. In contrast, the egalitarian and self-improvement attitudes that grew out of Australia's gold-rush period (1850s–1870s) served to create a stronger colonial work ethic. From the mid-1850s, the gradual expansion of the idea of the eight-hour workday was an effort (since Melbourne stonemasons won the 8-hour workday in 1856). Later, the introduction of the eight-hour workday (1910s) was an effort to improve the quality of working-class life by equally dividing the workday between work, leisure and rest.[93]

Chastity

Virginity and chastity were crucial social standards for women, but not for men. Many historians contend that the purpose of these standards was that marrying a virgin and having a chaste wife was how a man guaranteed his patrilineal legitimacy.[94] Assurance of bloodline remained the principal reason for these social conventions until syphilis began to spread across the world during the 15th century from the seaports of Europe.[95] With the spread of syphilis and other communicable diseases, abstinence from sexual activities outside the bounds of matrimony became more than social norm, it became a critical response to a severe and potentially deadly health issue. Virginity, chastity and abstinence became a means to limit the spread of these diseases.

While the surety of lineage and freedom from disease were reasons for working-class and middle-class compliance with this social convention, for the female convict population, the issues of chastity and monogamy came from a different set of reasons. Liston's research on the marriage of Parramatta's female convicts starts with Governor King's 1806 contention that female convicts at that time married as a means to get out of confinement.[96] More probable is that female convicts married or entered a de facto relationship for social, physical and sexual protection.[97] Marriage for female convicts was encouraged by the government to the point that in 1832 the advisory committee of the Female Factory placed advertisements to men "who are at all times disposed to favour the marriage of these Women persons in circumstances to maintain them honestly".[98] In other words, men could apply for a wife at the Parramatta Female Factory.[99] Not only did convict women marry for personal security, but they also married for the security of their offspring who were removed to the Orphan School when they were weaned and not returned until their mothers left the factory.[100]

Victorian values in literature

Much of what we know of the Victorian age comes from its literature. Woven into the fantasy, realism and sensationalism are social commentaries on class division, gender roles, industrialism and insights into childhood and health. Historian Margaret Marsh advises readers: "historians have become wary of advice literature and popular fiction as historical evidence, because used alone, they cannot help us to understand whether their strictures were followed".[101] Advice literature, such as Mrs Beeton's *Book of household management*

---

88 Haley 1979, 117.
89 Watson, Weir and Friend 2005, 4.
90 D.W. Brown 1987, 178.
91 Blair 1983, 10.
92 Franklin 1855.
93 Kimber and Love 2001, 1.

94 Mitchell 1981, xi; Harol 2006, 1.
95 V. Smith 2007, 1999–2000.
96 Hendriksen and Liston 2008, 32.
97 Salt 1984, 37–9.
98 *New South Wales Government Gazette* 30 May 1832, 111.
99 Hendriksen and Liston 2008, 45.
100 Salt 1984, 78.
101 Marsh 1990, 21.

(1861) went inside the middle-class Victorian home to demonstrate how it operated daily, while Miss Leslie's *The ladies' guide to true politeness and perfect manners or, Miss Leslie's behaviour book* (1864) supplied its reader with proper social protocols.[102] The *Australian etiquette, or the rules and usages of the best society in the Australasian colonies,* published in 1885, tailored Victorian etiquette for Australian society.[103]

The novels of popular Victorian authors, such as the Brontë sisters, Eliot and Dickens, created fictional characters who depicted the day-to-day social dynamics of middle-class society. Like the works of Jane Austen, the early 19th-century novels were commentaries on the lives of Britain's landed gentry. Social-class rigidity was a consistent theme in Austen's works, with her gentry-class characters doing nothing to earn their keep. In her novels (1811–1817), Austen wrote commentaries on her characters' appearance: she commented if a character had good teeth, well-groomed hair or wig and the latest style of fashionable clothing. More pertinent to this study, Austen wrote of medical conditions and ailments that afflicted the gentry. In Austen's published personal letters, she discusses various ailments suffered by family and friends, which suggests she drew on personal experiences for accounts of the medical conditions she wrote of in her novels.

In Victorian-era literature, the commentary shifted to the lives of the poor, working and middle classes. Novels of the Brontë sisters (1846–1854) depicted middle-class life in mid-Victorian-era England. Two of the most notable works by Charlotte Brontë, *Jane Eyre* and *Villette,* draw heavily on the author's personal life experiences and these novels depict working conditions for middle-class women employed through her lead characters. Where the sole purpose in life for Austen's gentrified heroines is to marry well, Brontë's middle-class heroines are powerful, clever and passionate in their struggles to find their place in society.

In Australia, James Tucker's 1844 novel *Ralph Rashleigh, or, the life of an exile* drew on personal experiences to portray the hierarchical convict class structure in colonial New South Wales. His symbolic narratives on the physical and spiritual degradation of convict labourers present an alternative portrayal of life in colonial New South Wales to that of colonial officials' memories or documents compiled in the *Historical Records of Australia.*[104]

Serial publications in magazines and journals facilitated the birth of the Victorian novel. Many of the noted novels of the day were first published in this format, including the works of Charles Dickens (1836–1870), Alexandre Dumas (1838–1870), Harriet Beecher Stowe (1843–1869), George Eliot (1859–1876) and Arthur Conan Doyle (1887–1929). The most successful of these authors was Charles Dickens, whose novels portrayed the human condition and social values in 19th-century Britain and, to some extent, the Australian colonies.

There are five distinct types of Victorian novels that have substantive portrayals of the working class: a cross-section of social classes; romance – usually the direct relationship between the gentry and the poor; non-romantic set entirely in a working-class environment; social propaganda – intended to alter the attitudes of the middle and upper classes towards the working class; and reform novels, such as temperance fiction that is explicitly directed at the working class.[105] The impact of temperance fiction is particularly pertinent to this study. The most influential writer of temperance fiction was Clara L. Balfour. Balfour was a temperance reformer turned author whose short novels were not of any literary acclaim. Her 28 novels were little more than thinly veiled temperance propaganda with titles such as *Toil and trust* and *Confessions of a decanter*.

As this chapter shows, the colonial class structure was not static. The many factors that contributed to the Australian ethos, foremost, are the resentment of the middle class by the working class, the self-improvement attitudes of radical "gold-rush" immigrants, the conservatism of the pastoralists and the influence of the members of the clergy through their role as magistrates in the colony. The evolution of social structure within the culture is crucial to understanding the influences Victorian values were able to assert. While fictional in content, Victorian literature is a source of information on class, social structure and health that enhances historical accounts. Next will be a detailed examination of archaeological and historical evidence of social status in Parramatta.

---

102 Beeton 1861; Miss Leslie 1864.
103 People's Publishing Company 1885.
104 Croft 1999, 15–16.

105 Keating 1971, 24–6.

Chapter 5
THE ARCHAEOLOGY OF SOCIAL CLASS

Historical archaeologists view class as a hierarchical scale through which people's lifestyles can be explained.[1] Marxist class analysts define class in terms of mechanisms of exploitation and domination.[2] Some sociologists define the general structure of class as the basic relations of a capitalist social order in the labour market.[3] Historian Linda Young goes further to contend that labour is the basic defining factor that separates working, middle and upper classes.[4] If labour is the basic factor of class, then power is how one class gains dominance over another. Power comes in many forms, including political, religious, monetary and social influences. One's ability to impose one's will on the behaviours of others determines the amount of power one person has over others, which influences both parties' social status.[5] Therefore, aligning an individual or family in the archaeological case study with a social class involves considering dynamics of Australian social structure and the tangible attributes that demonstrate the level of influence they have over others. Beaudry, Cook and Mrozowski compare and contrast theoretical approaches to the material expressions of culture and argue that "'cultural hegemony' represents the best approach to 'subsume complex processes of cultural change'".[6] They contend that the ever-shifting "prevailing consciousness" of members of social classes results in "competing ideologies centred around what they perceive to be in their own interest".[7] In archaeological scholarship, the detailed examination of class as a social construction is limited. Even more limited are archaeological constructs that examine social values. A study of the Victorian middle class in Brooklyn, New York, compares literature with the archaeological record to determine if middle-class behavioural conventions noted in literature can be verified in the archaeological records.[8] Young's middle-class culture study uses historic household goods and furnishing to identify common patterns of values, beliefs and behaviours.[9] Hayes' thesis identifies links between material culture and class by studying a Melbourne middle-class homestead.[10]

These works subscribe to a commonly held perception that social conventions are constructs through which people emulate their class superiors to socially elevate themselves. But Abercrombie and Turner's work on "dominant ideology theory" argues that examination of the position of subordinate classes shows they "rarely, or never, shared the ideology of the dominant".[11] Nonetheless, these values were more than just a set of etiquette rules. They were "proper" behaviours with moral connotations.[12] Adherence to these conventions demonstrated compliance that was critical to peer acceptance.

Seen archaeologically, the choice of quality goods demonstrates knowledge of "standards" and the capacity to acquire them.[13] Generally, archaeological scholarship recognises these standards' manifestation primarily in everyday life's material details. A monograph on a middle-class Melbourne household measured class by quality standards for matched sets of tableware and teaware, high-quality glassware, a large number of beverage bottles, expensive toys, personal items of luxury, matching toilet sets and medicine items.[14] An American study of 12 contiguous house lots in mid- to late 19th-century Brooklyn identifies material culture as active symbols that assist in assigning social class.[15] While the Brooklyn study emphasises matched tableware sets as indicators of middle-class status, it also looks beyond the typical domestic markers of social class to include introduced decorative motifs as class status symbols. A few archaeological studies have gone beyond these basic status indicators to examine the broader concepts that reflect class. One excellent example is Mrozowski's archaeological study that explores broader concepts with a comparative analysis of two American urban communities. Through case studies, it furthers the characteristics of class beyond consumer goods by the examination of yard-space usage and identifies aspirations of gentility through use patterns for medicinal plants, animal slaughter and pest control.[16]

---

1 Hayes 2014, 2.
2 Wright 2015, xi.
3 Connell and Irving 1980, 20.
4 Young 1988, 5.
5 Connell and Irving 1980, 17.
6 Beaudry, Cook and Mrozowski 1991, 280.
7 Beaudry, Cook and Mrozowski 1991, 280.
8 Fitts 1999.
9 Young 1988.
10 Hayes 2014.

11 Abercrombie and Turner 1978, 150.
12 Fitts 1999, 39.
13 Young 1988, 153.
14 Hayes 2014, 75.
15 Fitts 1999, 40.
16 Mrozowski 2006.

Table 5.1 House types identified for case-study sites.

Site number	Address	House type
1	4 George Street	Stone house
2	15 Macquarie Street	Timber house
3	45 Macquarie Street	Brick house
4–5	2 and 13–15 Taylor Street	Brick – semidetached dwellings
6	100 George Street	Weatherboard house (Halfpenny)
6	100 George Street	Stone house (Byrnes)
7	2 George Street	Weatherboard house
8	109 George Street	Brick house

Establishing social status for the Parramatta case-study households: archaeological evidence

The type of houses that residents built or purchased indicates their economic status more than their social status, yet these dwellings are contributing factors to socio-economic status assessments. Stone houses were the most expensive to construct, followed by brick, weatherboard and timber homes. Historical records and archaeological excavation identified these four basic house types among case-study sites (Table 5.1). Furthermore, house site locations within Parramatta's environmental setting are inclusive factors for socio-economic placement.

The typical archaeological paradigm for establishing socio-economic class is through the examination of artefact collections for high-quality goods as markers of class status. Presented here are a combined appraisal of the quality of goods with an interpretation of them as symbols of culture. There are four categories of artefacts that contributed to a comparative assessment of class for case-study sites: ceramic tableware, glass tableware, toys and personal grooming items. Glass and ceramic tableware are standard socio-economic indicators used by archaeologists to assess the status of a household. These categories of artefacts are typically the most abundant status indicator found in the artefact collections. Children's toys and personal grooming items represent a far lower percentage of case-study artefact collections but, depending on their quality or commercial value, they can be used as cultural symbols.

Analysis of the Parramatta ceramic tableware includes 1,229 refined earthenware and 277 porcelain vessels. Refined earthenware vessels were the norm in every 19th-century household. The quality of the vessels is the one factor that potentially contributes to a status assessment.[17] But the quality of the ceramic vessels was not included in the original analyses of the case-study sites' consultancy reports and precluded further analysis of this data.

Porcelain is often considered an indicator of social status, although this assumption must consider several factors. First, this comparative study limits porcelain vessels to European types because, from the 18th century, Chinese export porcelains were inexpensive utilitarian wares. Porcelain vessels from early convict-settlement households – sites 1, 6 (Halfpenny) and 7 – are mostly Chinese export porcelains, which are more indicative of trade networks than household status.[18]

Regardless of social status, most colonial households had porcelain tea services. Inviting guests to tea was one way a working-class lady could project an air of respectability. Domestic servants were typically expected in a 19th-century middle-class household; however, tea was traditionally served by the lady of the house. Therefore, the lack of servants in working-class households was not apparent to visitors.[19] Vessel forms common to a tea service include cups, saucers and small plates. As Table 5.2 shows, the majority of European porcelain vessels are teaware items.

In contrast, a porcelain dinner service is more indicative of a household's socio-economic status and how the household chose to entertain. The presence of such a service in site assemblages indicates a middle-class or middle-class gentry household.[20] Vessels associated with dinner service (plates, bowls, dishes, eggcups and a food service vessel lid) from the feature assemblages for sites 3, 4, 5, 6 and 7 suggest that these residents had a porcelain table service, as well as their tea service.

Glass tableware also contributes to socio-economic status assessment. The term "value" denotes the relative cost level to manufacture an item. Different stabilising materials are added to the flux, and the quality of these materials is indicative of cost, with lead representing the most expensive and soda lime the least expensive to produce. Decorative technique is another indicator of

---

17 Crook 2008.

18 Bach 1976, 48.
19 Harris 2005, 45; Lawrence and Davies 2010, 294.
20 Fitts 1998, 52; Lawrence and Davies 2010, 294.

Table 5.2 Relative frequencies of European porcelain vessel forms calculated for case-study sites.

Site number	Feature type	Feature number	Serving (%)	Cup (%)	Eggcup (%)	Mug (%)	Plate (%)	Plate, small (%)	Saucer (%)	Total minimum item count
2	Dam	10350						88.9	11.1	9
3	Well	650	5.0	62.0	8.3		0.8		24.0	121
5	Cistern	147		41.7		4.2	12.5	4.2	37.5	24
6	Cesspit	2206						100		4
6	Cesspit	2369						100		1
6	Cesspit	2370						100		1
6	Pit	1691						100		2
6	Well	2417	12.5					87.5		16
7	Cellar	3957		25.0			25.0	37.5	12.5	8
8	Pit	5073						100.		5

value with the more labour-intensive techniques assessed at a higher value. Cut decorations are achieved by skilled artisans, making their manufacture the most expensive decorative technique. Flint glassware or lesser-quality decorated glassware is considered a medium-valued item. Undecorated and press-moulded decorations, which could be mass produced, are the lowest-cost decorative technique. Therefore, a lead crystal glassware item with cut-glass decoration is ranked as the most expensive, while press-moulded soda-lime glassware is the least expensive. The combined factors of composition, manufacturing technique and decorative technique contributed to glass tableware's assignment to a ranked category based on value (Table 5.3).[21]

By the mid-19th century, children attained status worthy of their own material culture. Two categories of children's toys – marbles and toy dishes – were assessed as status indicators. There are three types of marbles in the case-study site assemblages (clay, stone and porcelain). Clay and stone types have been available for centuries to children of all social classes. Painted porcelain marbles became available by the 1800s and they were the most expensive type found in this study. Only glass German-spiral marbles were more expensive than painted porcelain marbles, but none was represented in the case-study collection.[22] Marbles have been advertised for sale in New South Wales since 1819, but no description was noted.[23] While there are 27 marbles recovered from case-study sites, porcelain marbles were recovered from only the McRoberts, the Byrnes and the Larkin household assemblages (sites 1, 6 and 7). Children's toy tea sets gain popularity during the first quarter of the 19th century, but most of these were refined white earthenware vessels. Vessels that comprise these toy tea sets are in the 15 Macquarie Street assemblage (site 2). In the 1840s, German porcelain toy tea sets were introduced at European exhibitions, but these items were only affordable to children in wealthier households.[24] Vessels from porcelain tea sets are in the site 3 assemblage.

Personal grooming items are a subset of personal hygiene and contribute to the assessment of personal health and social reforms, in particular their association with social status. With few exceptions, personal grooming items are common items available to all socio-economic classes. Fragrances were used by most case-study households, except for the Halfpenny household at site 6. Assessing the economic status of fragrances involves establishing their advertised cost, which requires identifying the fragrance's brand. Unfortunately, the only labelled bottles are high-priced (ranging from 1 shilling to £8 6 shilling), early 20th-century products from sites 4 and 5. A high-quality cutglass stopper for a perfume decanter and a tortoiseshell hair comb are in the site 1 assemblage.

The categories of artefact types discussed above are symbols of quality goods that typify what many historical archaeologists assign to higher socio-economic status. Blending the symbolism of these goods with the realities of a cultural setting allows for a more informed interpretation of their utility in assessing social status. Moreover, this interpretation presents just one measurement of social status. The following are summaries of case-study households and their status:[25]

---

21 Harris 2021, 211.
22 Carskadden and Gartley 1990, 57.
23 *Sydney Gazette and New South Wales Advertiser*, 21 August 1819.
24 Decker n.d.
25 Harris 2021, 178.

Table 5.3 Relative frequencies of glass tableware by quality established for case-study sites.

Site number	Address	Feature type	Feature number	High value (%)	Medium value (%)	Low value (%)	Total Minimum item count
1	4 George St	Cesspit	6024	33.3	44.4	22.2	9
1	4 George St	Cesspit	6039	100			1
2	15 Macquarie St	Dam	10350		66.7	33.3	6
3	45 Macquarie St	Well	650	30.4	17.4	52.2	23
4	2 Taylor St	Cistern	4702		100		9
5	13–15 Taylor St	Cistern	147		100		2
6	100 George St	Cesspit	2206		57.1	42.9	7
6	100 George St	Cesspit	2369	42.9	14.3	42.9	7
6	100 George St	Cesspit	2370	71.4		28.6	7
6	100 George St	Well	2417	28.6	28.6	42.9	7
7	2 George St	Cellar	3957	14.3	71.4	14.3	7
8	109 George St	Pit	5073	40.0	40.0	20.0	5

- Site 1 – the McRoberts family lived in a stone house. There is no archaeological evidence that they owned a porcelain teaware service. The majority of their ceramic tableware was refined earthenware (creamware, pearlware and whiteware), but also included Chinese export porcelain. Their table was set with mostly high- and medium-valued glass tableware. The McRoberts children played with widely affordable clay and stone marbles and high-value porcelain toy marbles. The lady of the house owned a cutglass perfume decanter and a costly tortoiseshell hair comb. Collectively, these artefact types are consistent with a strong middle-class status.
- Site 2 – the Noble household lived in a timber-constructed house. They owned a porcelain teaware service. Their table was set with medium- to low-value glass tableware. The Noble children played with widely affordable clay marbles and an earthenware teaware set. The collective consideration of these artefact types is consistent with a working-class status.
- Site 3 – the Walker and Sweeney families lived in a brick house. They owned a porcelain teaware service that included a teapot. Their table was set with both earthenware and porcelain dinnerware and high- and low-valued glass tableware. The children played with widely affordable clay and stone marbles, and also had a high-value porcelain toy teaware set. The collective consideration of these artefact types is consistent with a strong middle-class status.
- Sites 4–5 – The assemblages for these tenanted brick semidetached dwellings included similar class-related markers. At both dwellings, the tables were set with medium-valued glass tableware and, by the early 20th century, both used high-value fragrances. No porcelain teaware was recovered from Site 4, but porcelain teaware and dinnerware was used by the tenants of Site 5. The collective consideration of these artefact types is consistent with a middle-class standing.
- Site 6 – There were two occupations of this site. Thomas Halfpenny lived in a weatherboard house. He owned a porcelain teaware set. His tableware was set with mostly undecorated creamware, pearlware and Chinese export porcelain vessels. No glass tableware was found in this assemblage. The collective consideration of these artefact types is consistent with a working-class status. Three generations of the Byrnes family lived in a two-storey stone house. They owned a porcelain teaware service. Their table was set with both earthenware and porcelain dinnerware and all values of glass tableware. The children played with clay and porcelain marbles. The collective consideration of these artefact types is consistent with a middle-class standing.
- Site 7 – The Larkin family lived in a weatherboard house. They owned a porcelain teaware set. The Larkins' table was set with mostly refined earthenware (creamware, pearlware and whiteware), but they also used Chinese export porcelain (33 per cent). Their table was set with mostly medium-value glass tableware and there is one porcelain dinner plate in the assemblage. The children played with clay, stone and porcelain marbles. The collective consideration

5 The archaeology of social class

Table 5.4 Summary information for the status and class of residents in the case study.

Site number	Name	Status	Class	Artefact date range
1	James McRoberts	free settler	middle	1820–60
2	John Noble	convict/ticket-of-leave	working	1823–41
3	John Walker	Australian born	middle	1860–80
3	George Sweeney	Australian born	middle	1860–90
4	Henry Byrnes	Australian born	middle	1890s–1920
5	Tenanted	various	middle	1890–1930
6	Thomas Halfpenny	ex-marine/free settler	working	1790–1830
6	Byrnes Family	Australian born	middle/gentry	1840–1930
7	Samuel Larkin	emancipist	working	1810–40s
8	Hassall Family	free settler	middle/gentry	1820–80

of these artefact types is inconclusive and suggests a marginal middle-class standing.
- Site 8 – The Hassalls' brick two-storey house was home to three generations of the family. They owned a porcelain teaware set. Their table was set with mostly matched transfer-printed earthenware ceramic tableware, and high- to medium-valued glass tableware. The collective consideration of these artefact types is consistent with a middle-class standing.

So, in conclusion, the range of social status indicators, such as house types and status markers, further our knowledge of the socio-economic status aspirations of households in the case study.

Establishing social status for the Parramatta case-study households: documentary evidence

For each site, an individual or individuals were identified for the timeframe of the dated, sealed deposit or deposits used in the case study. In most instances, identification of the individuals was taken from historical documentation included in heritage consultancy reports, which is often comprised of basic statistics such as date of occupancy and occupation. While gender and ethnicity are not a focus here, any documented data on these topics is considered. Supplementary research involved various sources, including Parramatta histories, online biographies, archived newspaper articles, notices and advertisements. Additional research allowed the compilation of details regarding religious affiliations, civic involvement and social activities. Furthermore, identifying key artefact types discussed above provides tangible evidence contributing to social-class assignment. The collective data for each individual are assessed to determine their social-class placement in Victorian society. Such assessments are subjective due to limitations of available facts and the author's 21st-century perception used to interpret those facts. The approach taken was to collect the tangible data and determine the degree of influence these factors afforded one person over others (exploitation or domination).

This assessment determined that there was representation from the working class, the middle class and the middle-class gentry. Table 5.4 provides a summary for individuals with data used to assess their class status. The summaries below are based on biographical information included in the appendix.

There are three individuals whose lives demonstrate working-class attributes:

- Site 2 – John Noble, who lived at 15 Macquarie Street (1820s–40s), was working class. He was a repeat offender convict. Noble was an illiterate baker. No accounts of civic or benevolent activities were associated with him.
- Site 6 – Thomas Halfpenny lived at 100 George Street (1804–10). He was working class. An ex-marine from the First Fleet, Halfpenny married convict Catherine Wilmot. He engaged in the grain trade and was a boat operator for Ann Mash's passenger boat service to Parramatta.[26] In 1810, he died and the auction notice for the property listed a five-bedroom shingled and weatherboard house.[27]
- Site 7 – Samuel Larkin lived at 2 George Street (1814–38). His social status was working class. His home was a convict cottage. He was literate and promotable, but his questionable use of his government position to acquire property would not have found favour in the middle class, nor would his activism for emancipist property rights. There are no accounts of any civic or benevolent activities associated with Larkin. Finally, Larkin was first and foremost an ex-convict, which was a barrier to social acceptance by the middle class.

---
26 McClymont 2014.
27 Kass 2002, 5.

Table 5.5 Summary of occupations and activities identified for middle-class residents of Taylor Street.

Site number	Occupant	Address	Occupation	Civic activities	Social activities	Occupancy date
	F. Wickham	3 Taylor St	Railway Accountant	Election poll clerk Auditor Civic Building Society	Sec. cricket club Churchwarden	1875–92
4	Henry Byrnes	2 Taylor St	Captain – Parramatta Corps	Magistrate Commission to Supreme Court	Churchwarden	1875–92
4	Ellen Curling	2 Taylor St	Medical practitioner		Church volunteer	1878
	L.A. Simpson	9 Taylor St	Dentist	Alderman/mayor		1899–1922
	F. Pearson	Taylor St	Veterinary surgeon			1920–1921
	F.J. Thomas	Taylor St	Accountant	Secretary Parramatta Progress Association		1909
	F. Todhunter	11 Taylor St	Lawyer			1908
	F. MacQueen	Taylor St	Bank officer	Parramatta Hospital committee	Active church member Bowling club Chess club	1902

There are three individual landowners from the case study sites and eight tenants from five Taylor Street properties (Table 5.5) whose lives demonstrate middle-class attributes:

- Site 1 – James McRoberts lived at 4 George Street (1846–60). His social status was middle class. He was a free settler who first served in the respectable position of the jailer in Parramatta. While his home was acquired through marriage, his successful business endeavours led to the purchase of one of Parramatta's most successful pubs. His household included servants, a standard in a middle-class home. Finally, McRoberts' benevolent and religious activities in the community were exemplars of Victorian values.
- Site 3 – John Walker lived at 45 Macquarie Street (1823–70s). He was a marginal middle-class individual. A native-born son of an unwed convict, Walker was literate and a wheelwright by trade and also an inspector for the slaughterhouses in Parramatta. He received a town grant for the property at 45 Macquarie Street after he had built a substantial brick house and several outbuildings. There are no accounts of Walker's involvement with civic and benevolent organisations or of his religious affiliation.
- Site 3 – Samuel George Valentine Sweeney lived at 45 Macquarie Street (1879–86). He was middle class. He worked in the family business as a coachbuilder. Sweeney was civic-minded and was elected alderman for Marsden Ward, Parramatta, in 1882.[28]
- Sites 4–5 – The five properties on the west side of Taylor Street between D'Arcy and Macquarie streets were all owned and tenanted by George Coates. Historical records indicate that many of the residents (1875–1920) were literate and prosperous middle-class professionals and, as Table 5.5 shows, many were involved in civic and social activities.

The two semidetached houses (sites 4 and 5), erected by George Coates in the 1870s, were located on higher ground (more than 12 metres above sea level) and had no issues with drainage or severe mould. With their prominent preferred position, these dwellings were built on the eastern extent of D'Arcy Wentworth's subdivided estate. Wentworth was a highly regarded and influential government official in the late 18th century. In 1812, he received a 32-acre land grant in Parramatta on which he constructed Woodhouse, a fine manor house. These dwellings were tenanted by mostly middle-class professionals who could afford the rental costs in this desirable neighbourhood (Table 5.5).

There are two affluent families whose social status ranked above middle class. Termed here as middle-class gentry, each of these families was a pillar of the community, each in a different way:

---

28 *Australian Town and Country Journal* 11 February 1882, 15.

- Site 6 – The Byrnes family lived at 100 George Street (1830–1952). The family was more than just middle class; they were quasi-gentry. William Byrnes (1809–1891) was born in Sydney to James Byrnes, a pensioner of the 8th Regiment. William and his brother James carried on extensive businesses as general merchants, including a wine and spirits wholesale warehouse, a woollen mill and flour mill in Parramatta. At various times in his life, William served as postmaster at Parramatta, a trustee of the Parramatta Savings Bank, was a district magistrate and served on the Legislative Council from 1857. He was also a Freemason[29]

  Byrnes built a Georgian manor on George and Charles streets' north-east corner in the 1830s where his spinster daughters, Emmeline and Marian, lived most of their lives. A third Byrnes sister, Ann Pringle (widowed), resumed her place in the Byrnes household in 1921 along with her daughter, Alice Maud Hogarth Pringle, who lived in the family home until her death at the age of 86 in 1952

  Emmeline Byrnes' social outings were often noted in newspaper accounts.[30] At her death in 1921 Miss Emmeline Pringle's estate was worth £16,395 (AUD $1.6 million in 2023). Marian Byrnes was also very socially active in her church and had a particular interest in politics.[31] For several social occasions, her fashionable attire was noted in newspaper society columns.[32]

- Site 8 – Rowland Hassall's family lived at 109 George Street (1804–1870s). They were middle-class gentry. In 1804, Hassall's 1799 lease was converted to a land grant, and he built a home with bricks he imported from Britain. The same year Hassall had informally acquired adjacent leases, expanding his property to 5.5 acres, upon which he developed a complex including gardens and a dairy. Rowland Hassall also opened a store at this location, which is thought to be the first private business in Parramatta.[33] By 1808 Hassall had acquired grants to 1,300 acres in various locations from Dundas district to Camden, on which he ran his sheep and those of other flockmasters.[34] In 1814, he was appointed superintendent of government stock.[35]

  Hassall was best known for his ministry. He was an itinerant preacher, holding services for various Protestant congregations throughout the district. In Parramatta, he held Sunday and Friday services in his barn. When Hassall died in 1830, his family carried on his business interests and ministry.

While social class was a criterion for site selection, the residents' backgrounds (that is, heritage, convict or free settler, and family history) were not a factor. But their histories demonstrate a diversity in heritage and how they came to live in Parramatta. Some were Australian-born, but others came to the colony as convicts or free settlers. Australian-born residents were children of convicts, free settlers and retired military. Some immigrated on their own, while others came with their families.

The fluidity and mobility of social classes are also noted for the residents. Class mobility is indicated for two residents (sites 1 and 3) who were well placed in much-needed trade occupations that are traditionally working-class vocations. Moreover, McRoberts (site 1) demonstrated a strong work ethic and community involvement, indicating upward mobility in his social status. Conversely, neither of the emancipated convicts bettered their social status through involvement in civic or religious affiliations (sites 2 and 7). By the second generation, the mobility of the middle-class gentry residents was stagnant because, in the late 19th-century colonial culture, there was no upper class to which they could aspire. Finally, the late 19th-century residents on Taylor Street exemplify an emerging group of educated middle-class professionals.

The dynamic in the Australian class structure is power, which is influenced by political, religious, monetary and social factors. The ability of one social class to impose its social values on another to stimulate change is apparent in 19th-century Parramatta, especially in the promotion of Victorian values held by the middle class. The Parramatta archaeology provides evidence for the aspiration of all classes to adhere to these values through the identification of social markers, such as where they lived and the quality of their commercial goods. In the next chapter, these markers are taken together to form a foundation for an examination of the extent Victorian values influenced attitudes towards health within the social classes.

---

29 *Evening News* 26 October 1891, 5.
30 *Evening News* 16 August 1902, 4.
31 *Cumberland Argus and Fruitgrowers Advocate* 4 September 1897, 12; *The Methodist* 15 March 1930, 20.
32 *Cumberland Argus and Fruitgrowers Advocate* 9 September 1911, 11.
33 *Cumberland Argus and Fruitgrowers Advocate* 7 February 1928, 6.
34 Gunson 1966.
35 Binney 2005, 64.

Chapter 6
THE HISTORY OF COLONIAL MEDICINE, PUBLIC HEALTH AND ENVIRONMENTAL REFORM

This chapter starts with a review of the relevant medical history sources. It outlines the public health issues and private health concerns in early colonial Australia, which can be summarised as bleak for all due to poor nutrition, exacerbated by excessive drinking for many. The next section of this chapter examines the historical documentation and archaeological evidence for public health initiatives and environmental reforms in 19th-century Parramatta.

Relevant medical history sources

This work separates medicine into two basic categories: orthodox medicine and traditional health care. Orthodox (or allopathic) medicine treats symptoms and diseases with compounded or prescription drugs and invasive surgery. Bynum's thesis contends that orthodox medicine is the product of 19th-century society.[1] Traditional health care describes medical treatments that rely on long-established knowledge and skills, akin to modern-day homeopathic or naturopathic medicine, with origins that pre-date the science of orthodox medical practices.[2] In her alternative history of Australian medicine, Martyr states that traditional medicine was the standard medical treatment practised by most individuals in Australia's Georgian and Victorian eras.[3]

The language of medical history

Medical history is often influenced by the Whiggism theory, which perceives modern medicine's development as resulting from a natural progression towards the ideas and institutions of the age. Consequently, medical historians tend to shape the history of medicine using current definitions and understanding ("presentism"), or they view ideas or disciplines as basically the same in all ages ("essentialism").[4] When reading published and unpublished historical accounts of colonial New South Wales, one must consider the perceptions and conscious and unconscious biases that influenced the author, deriving information from those works with consideration for the cultural (and often ethnocentric) context in which they were written.

Language and linguistics have a crucial role in interpreting historical and technical medical terminology found in historical documents. Here, I take a cautious and analytical approach to the recognition and interpretation of the medical terminology encountered in contemporary documents, allowing that this changed and evolved over the 112 years that fall within the scope of this study and the 120 years that followed. Table 6.1 clarifies terms used for medical practitioners as they were defined during the colonial era.

There is also a plethora of medical terminologies that historically had different meanings. For the most part, these terms do not appear within the pages of this publication. Their historical definition (Table 6.1) is crucial to the analytical classification of artefact types. For example, the simplest term, like the use of the word "cordial" in a historic medical document, can be misleading. "Cordial" was historically a class of invigorating heart stimulants, not the non-alcoholic fruit-flavoured concentrate popular in Australia since the 1900s.[5]

Another factor when consulting historical documents is the language used by one segment of society to describe another. Attention must be paid to written accounts wherein authority figures discuss their subordinates.[6] An example of one such pattern can be seen in misogynistic accounts written by male settlers or men in positions of authority about female convicts, describing them all as "whores".[7] The descriptors they used regarding the female convicts' actions were not because the women in question were prostitutes, but rather that they drank, smoked, used foul language, dressed in men's clothing and dared to look a gentleman in the eye, all because as Oxley succinctly states: "Dissatisfaction with the women was expressed in sexual terminology: they became whores, a metaphorical device distilling all the features that were the obverse of what became the Victorian feminine ideal".[8] This statement underpins just one aspect of Victorian values with regard to differences in social-class practices and the notion of "respectability".

Public and personal health

In the 1830s and 1840s, English barrister Edwin Chadwick set forth concepts, terms and standards for public health that were progressively introduced throughout the 19th century. Chadwick redefined the

---

1 Bynum 1994, xi.
2 Martyr 2002.
3 Martyr 2002.
4 Ferngren 2014, 13–14.

5 Ritter 1917, 828.
6 Cook 2008, 217.
7 Oxley 1996, 203.
8 Oxley 1996, 203.

Table 6.1 A list of defined terms used for medical practitioners.

Term	Historic definition
Barber	A barber-surgeon was akin to the 21st-century "general practitioner", who consulted for a range of ailments from lancing boils to bloodletting and amputations.
Surgeon	Orthodox-trained medical practitioners serving in military units; the designation was not limited to physicians who perform invasive surgery. Surgeons more frequently received their training through an apprenticeship.
Midwife	Women experienced in the natural delivery of babies, who were trained through an apprenticeship, often at the side of their mothers or older female family members.
man-midwife	Man-midwives required no certification beyond their medical credentials as a surgeon or apothecary. They were predecessors to modern-day obstetricians.
Wise woman	Female herbalists and midwives.
Medical practitioner	Anyone working as a biomedical healer.
Apothecary	Preparer of physicians' prescriptions and a predecessor to compounding chemists.
Bonesetter	Set broken bones and dislocated joints as well as repairing ruptures.
Empiric	A person who, in medicine or other sciences, relies solely on observation and experiment.
Physician	Men medically educated at institutions of higher learning, with all of their studies reliant on lectures and the reading of written works with minimal hands-on experience before entering their profession.

problem of the people's health as one of engineering: the question of removing environmental filth, which was the cause of ill health and premature death in cities. Inspired by Chadwick, American John Griscom believed sanitary improvement to be linked to the moral uplift of the poor. His 1844 report to the New York City Health Department documented the vast numbers of illness and mortality that could have been prevented by cost-effective government public health action.[9]

Personal health is a diverse topic comprised of many overlapping and entwined themes relating to medicine, nutrition, hygiene, social class and colonial convictism. Through medical archaeology approaches, Hsu proposes that artefact-based contextual studies can contribute information not available through literature.[10] Unfortunately, as Baker and Carr assert, there are limited archaeological interpretive methods for understanding medicine.[11] Therefore, understanding the evolution from traditional to orthodox health care requires examining relevant historical research on health care. This begins with background research in Britain, such as Porter and Wear, who are two of many medical historians of 16th-century to 19th-century medicine in Britain.[12] It continues with Evans', Lewis' and Hagger's overviews of colonial health and medicine,[13] while Brown's volume on medical practice in "Old Parramatta" contributes a wealth of information on health care and medical practitioners in Parramatta from its earliest days.[14] Green and Cromwell's work on friendly societies discusses how the late-19th-century friendly societies came together to form medical institutes that provided affordable health care, such as the Parramatta and District United Friendly Societies' Medical and Dispensing Institute.[15]

The investigation of public and personal health includes examining prevalent illnesses and diseases and available medical treatments. Research on infant health and mortality discusses the first generation of colonists and how dysentery, thrush and respiratory diseases were the most life-threatening ailments affecting children. Gandevia's research on children's health identifies marasmus (malnutrition) as a major cause of juvenile death in early colonial times. However, Maxwell-Stewart's study on colonial health suggests that the nutrition of children born in the colony of British free immigrants and convicts was much improved over that afforded their parents during their own formative years. Sprenger's research attributes advancements in orthodox medicine for the drop in infant mortality as the 19th century progressed.[16]

Inadequate nutrition was a key factor of ill health in the early colony. Clements' research on nutrition in Australia reports on the lack of good nutrition in early colonial days. It details the changes that progressively brought about healthier diets throughout the 19th century.[17] Researchers

---

9 Lewis 2014, 7–11; Peterson 1979, 86.
10 Hsu 2002, 16.
11 Baker and Carr 2002, vii.
12 Porter 1993.
13 Evans 1983; Hagger 1979; Lewis 2014.
14 K.M. Brown 1937.
15 Green and Cromwell 1984, 97–8.
16 Gandevia 1978; Lewis 2014, 201; Maxwell-Stewart 2006; Sprenger 2012, 13.
17 Clements 1986.

and historians fail to note that high alcohol consumption (four times that of Britain) in early colonial times contributed to widespread thiamine deficiencies.[18] Lewis and Dingle present thorough statistical representations of Australian alcohol consumption throughout the Victorian era. They discuss the state of policies and the economy since they affected the cost and availability of alcohol, but they do not address the extent to which health or social aspects were affected by consumption patterns.[19] But research also indicates that, as early as the mid-17th century, medical practitioners recognised that excess drinking was associated with moral and physical ills.[20]

Personal health in 19th-century Australia

Personal health relates to the wellbeing of individuals. A society promotes wellbeing through developing systems for proactive and reactive health care; proactive health care is achieved through healthy lifestyle patterns while reactive health care is the treatment of mental and physical illnesses.

A natural prelude to discussing personal health concerns in Parramatta is a synopsis of the general state of health care in 19th-century Australia. For the first 50 years of European settlement in Australia (1788–1830s), medical care for convicts and free settlers was available free of charge from surgeons of the Colonial Medical Service.[21] Availability depended on factors such as proximity to settlements where medical attention could be obtained and the availability of the government-appointed medical practitioners. From the beginning of Parramatta's settlement, most of the early government-appointed medical practitioners were more interested in agricultural pursuits than their official duties of care and treatment of the convict and free settlers.[22] This rudimentary healthcare system left most to their own resources for medical care.

Assessing the general health of the colonial population is fraught with difficulties. Maxwell-Stewart contends that, despite the complexity of accounting for all factors affecting an individual's wellbeing, "height indices remain one of the best available comparative measures for assessing the well-being of populations".[23] In fact, height was one of the factors used to estimate a convict's health when selecting who was to be transported.[24] Australia's "cornstalk" generation consists of the colonially born children in the first half of the 19th century with at least one convict parent, so-called because they were noticeably taller than their parents.[25] The mortality rate during the first few years of colonisation was high. The burials of perinates, recovered during archaeological investigations in the grounds of Parramatta Hospital, are indicative of the stillborn and miscarriage problems that complicated childbirth during the first quarter of the 19th century. The children who survived benefited from the isolation of the colony from most of the world. This isolation resulted in the absence of common childhood infections until the 1830s.[26]

To comprehend personal health care in the 19th century, one must understand medical practices of the previous centuries, practices that had changed little for centuries. Prior to the 19th century, plant, animal, and mineral remedies were the basis for primary treatments. Traditionally, health care was attended to in a family setting. Home health care evolved over the millennia with recipes for traditional herbal and mineral-based remedies passed down, mostly among women, as part of herbal medicine's folk culture. The family medicine chest was stocked with plants and minerals collected from the provincial landscape that were ingredients needed to prepare these recipes.[27]

In the mid-18th century, the dawn of the British Industrial Revolution witnessed a shift from an agrarian society to a more urbanised society. Families now found themselves cut off from their traditional herbal medicine roots. No longer did they have access to the raw materials to prepare their recipes, and they were also distanced from the wise family healers who were well versed in the use of these remedies. These transplanted people in the newly created urban setting created new consumers, resulting in the rapidly developing patent and proprietary medicine market. At this time, consumer confidence in orthodox medical practitioners was very low, as prior to 19th-century advancements in orthodox medicine, the main prescribed treatments for all ailments were bloodletting, blistering and cupping.

Similar to 18th-century health care, the early 19th-century lay medical practice was centred on the family as the first source of treatment. However, colonial transportation and immigration often meant the absence of a family structure, and left unknowledgeable patients to consult the local apothecary, who often prescribed whatever patent medicine was available in his shop.

Public health and environmental reforms in colonial Parramatta

Environmental health involves those aspects of public health concerned with the factors, circumstances and conditions in the environment or surroundings of humans that can exert an influence on health and wellbeing.[28]

---

18 Blocker, Fahey and Tyrrell 2003, 79.
19 Dingle 1980; Lewis 1992.
20 Allen 2013; Lewis 1992, 98.
21 Lewis 2014, 201.
22 K.M. Brown 1937, 2.
23 Maxwell-Stewart 2006, 40–1.
24 Oxley 1996, 112.
25 Maxwell-Stewart 2006, 40–1.

26 Lewis 2014, 201.
27 Wear 2000, 21.
28 Smith, Whiley and Ross 2021.

Table 6.2 Weekly food rations were provided to all settlers based on the First Fleet Rations. Source: *Historical Records of New South Wales*, 5 July 1788, I, ii: 143.

Seamen	7 lbs bread/biscuit, 4 lbs beef, 2 lbs pork, 2 pints peas, 3 pints oatmeal, 8 ozs butter, 12 ozs cheese and 7 gallons beer.
Male convicts	7 lbs bread or flour, 7 lbs beef or 4 lbs pork, 3 pints peas, 6 ozs butter and 1 lb flour or half lb rice.
Female convicts	Two-thirds of the male convict rations.
Reduced rations	Initial weekly rations were reduced as food became scarce, to 2 lbs salt pork, 2 1/2 lbs flour and 2 lb rice for adults by mid-1790.

> *Parramatta, like most settlements, had both areas of good, healthy environmental settings and poor, unhealthy ones. Shortly after arriving in Parramatta in 1799, Reverend Rowland Hassall received a 14-year lease on a one-acre lot on high ground – a natural alluvial terrace with a gentle slope – and by 1804, he built a brick home. There are several key facts packed into that statement. First, Hassall arrived in Parramatta as a respected free immigrant of middle-class standing. Secondly, soon after arrival, he received a land grant. Thirdly, the land grant was for an allotment on a high, well-drained site. And finally, he built a substantial home on the property. The location of his land grant most likely reflected his social status and his ability to construct a sturdy home. This suggests that status was a factor in the assignment of land grants, and individuals of higher status and wealth were afforded allotments in more environmentally healthy locations. Many of the public health issues and environmental reforms that took place in 19th-century Parramatta dealt not with issues affecting those residing on the higher elevations but rather the individuals living in the boggy areas of the settlement.*

Assessing the relationship of colonial public health to the environmental reforms developed to promote collective wellbeing is key to understanding the reasons for public initiatives. These initiatives are best demonstrated through medical anthropology and ecology approaches. But consideration must also be afforded to the reactionary cultural factors and the political-economic systems that developed to handle these issues.

Colonial public health: historical sources

Nutrition

Nutrition is the relationship between food supply, dietetics (the effect of diet on health) and health. It affects both public and personal health issues, and for continuity, all elements of nutrition are presented together in the following discussion of the Parramatta samples. Not included are archaeological analysis results for food remains due to inconsistent field approaches to the collection, identification and analysis of these materials. For most sites, faunal remains were collected, retained and catalogued and for all but a few sites these remains were analysed. In most instances, macro-flora food remains, such as nuts, seeds and stones (pits), were subject to a rudimentary analysis. Nevertheless, methodological approaches were insufficient to achieve a comprehensive excavated collection for the recovery of smaller macro-flora, such as berry and grape seeds. Analysed pollen samples exist for only two sites featured in the case study. The interpretation of food-related pollens is discussed below.

Food supply was a critical public health concern at the time of first settlement. Early settlers were sustained mostly on rations from the government stores because the land in Sydney's vicinity was not suitable for growing crops. The initial weekly ration for all members of the First Fleet was based on naval regulations (Table 6.2). Due to food scarcity, rations were reduced to two-thirds in 1789.[29]

Nutritional deficiencies in this Australian diet affected the health of early settlers, yet despite extreme provision shortages at no stage was the early colony literally starving.[30] Vitamin C deficiencies resulted in rampant scurvy that was treated with locally sourced berries. There were several wholesome local native plants, including wild celery, spinach, figs, cherries and samphire that grew on the heaths, and convicts and officers alike supplemented their diet by collecting these native foods.[31] Regrettably, all accounts were reported by officers, such as Governor Phillip, Captain Tench and Surgeon Worgan, and not by the convicts who laboured ten to 12 hours per day, six days per week, with little time to forage for new food sources. Most settlers (convict or free) were just struggling to survive in this new land with unfamiliar vegetation and climate.

Thiamine (vitamin B1) deficiency, also termed beriberi, is characterised by muscle weakness and atrophy, blurred vision and, in extreme cases, heart failure. This dietary deficiency should have been almost non-existent among early European settlers in Australia, due to their heavy reliance on wheat-based food sources and flour milling methods that produced "wholemeal" flour, which retains

---

29 Polya 2001, 1.
30 Gandevia 1975, 6.
31 Barton 1989, 276; Karskens 2010, 273.

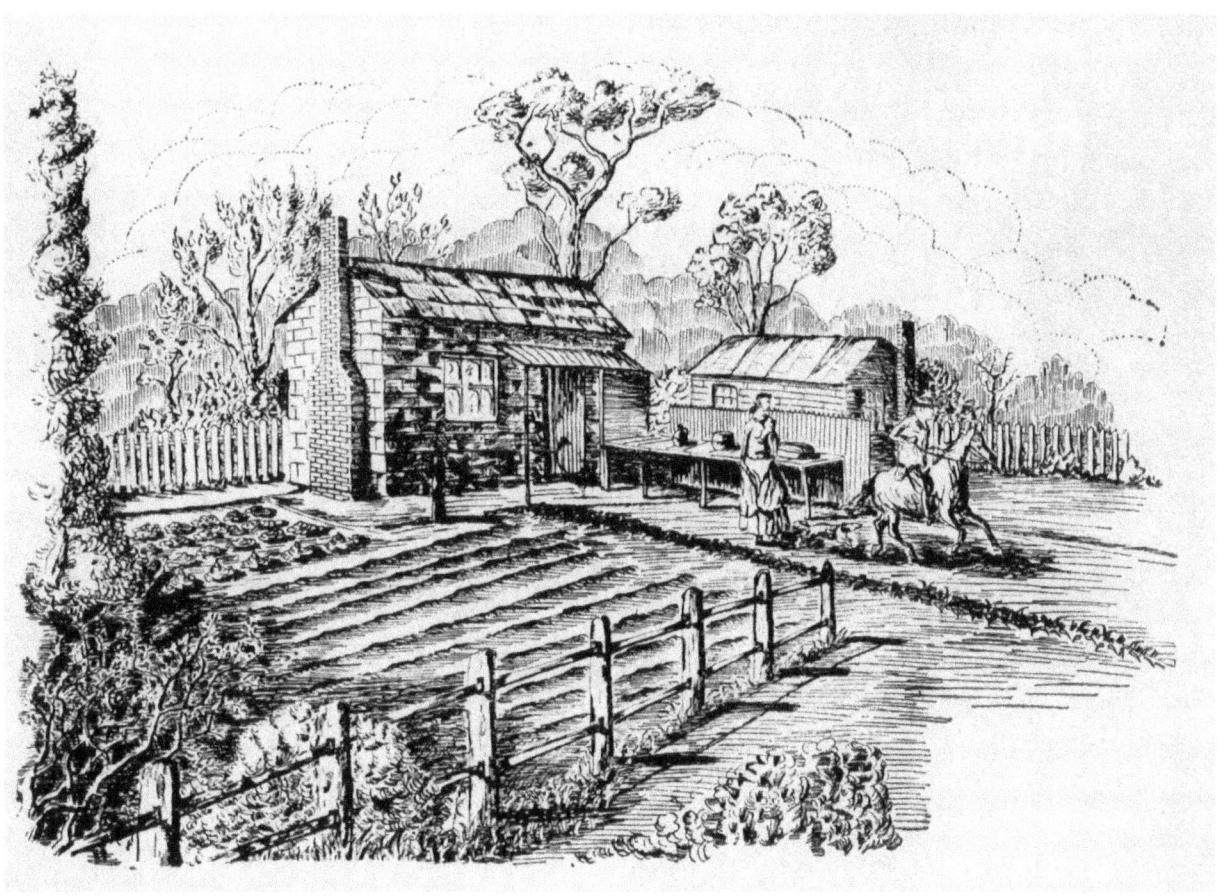

Figure 6.1 Reconstructed 1800s sketch showing a cottage and garden, Barrack Lane, Parramatta. Source: Rivett 1961, 47.

much of its thiamine. It should be noted that not all nutritional deficiencies resulted from diet. Thiamine deficiency is also associated with chronic alcoholism, a common problem in the early settlement.[32]

Rickets is a softening of bones due to lack of calcium and phosphorus. Vitamin D helps the body absorb these minerals. Vitamin D deficiency usually results from a lack of adequate sunlight which was a problem for only a small sector of the New South Wales population, affecting the housebound, the infirm, the physically impaired and the infants of the poor.

As the colony became settled and the initial food crisis passed, nutritional deficiencies lessened. Meal patterns began to realign with the colonists' lifestyles and social status brought with them to the colony, and, thus, for many, nutrition became a personal health concern. For many convicts, their weekly rations were nutritionally superior to the working-class diet they had left behind in Britain. As Dr Philip Muskett, Surgeon Superintendent to the New South Wales Government (1883), would later comment: "these Australian food habits are characterised by a preponderance of meat diet and a corresponding neglect of vegetable products", a dietary pattern that was common until the mid-20th century.[33]

Convicts and military personnel from a middle-class background took advantage of the gardens around their cottages to grow vegetables. Illustrations of early Parramatta show some cottages with fruit trees and vegetable gardens, but little is written about what residents grew in their cottage gardens and served at their dinner tables (Figure 6.1). Fortunately, a 2008 city-wide pollen study in Parramatta from four 19th-century archaeological sites identified fossil pollens for cereals and a variety of vegetables (cabbage or turnip, carrot or celery, and peas), fruits (strawberry) and fruit trees (peach, plum, cherry, apple, pear and fig).[34]

Government officials, many from the lower gentry of British society, were accustomed to a diet rich with fruits and vegetables. They were quick to establish their own gardens in the colony.[35] In 1795, Elizabeth Macarthur, the wife of colonial secretary and pastoralist John Macarthur, wrote of almond, pear and apple trees on her Parramatta property, Elizabeth Farm. After they arrived in 1800, Governor King's wife Anna supervised the creation of

---

32 Blocker, Fahey and Tyrrell 2003, 79.

33 Clements 1986, 34.
34 MacPhail and Casey 2008, 54.
35 Clements 1986, 34.

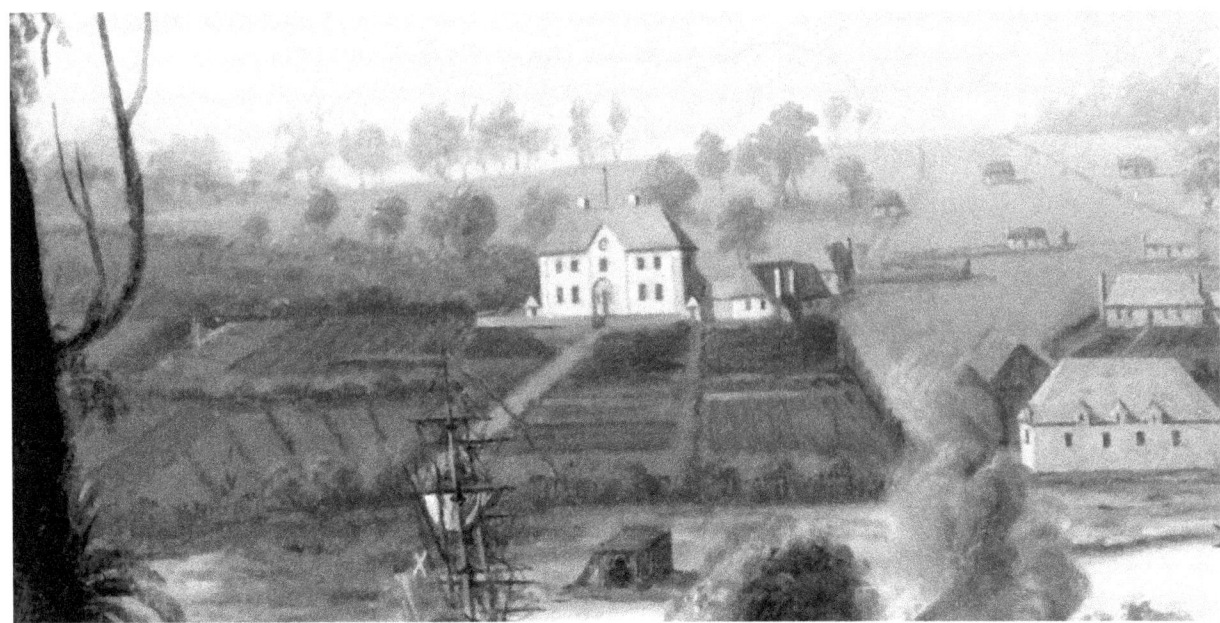

Figure 6.2 A view showing the first, early 19th-century Government House, Sydney, and its vegetable gardens. Source: State Library of New South Wales (a795001/ DG 60).

large geometrically laid-out vegetable gardens at First Government House in Sydney (Figure 6.2).[36]

During the earliest period of settlement, the government's single function was the operation of a self-sustaining jail, where convict labour produced food for the colony.[37] Much is written about crops grown by the early government initiatives at Parramatta during early colonial times.[38] Grains, such as wheat, barley and maize, were the initial focus as they were a source of the meal for bread.[39] Private crop production, which began in the 1790s, gradually increased the volume and variety of available crops. The establishment of regional sheep and cattle stations by pastoralists such as John Macarthur secured a ready supply of inexpensive meat. Dairies also operated from the early 1790s, with their butter and cheese sold at Parramatta's markets.[40] After 1803, a limited supply of imported foods, such as cheeses, hams and pickles, arrived from Britain and made their way into the Parramatta market.[41] The establishment of Parramatta's Market Place in 1813, with its weekly markets and semi-annual fairs, ensured the availability of these products to all the town's residents.[42] The 1830s establishment of market gardens by European settlers in New South Wales added a ready supply of produce to the marketplaces.[43] Market gardens have continued as a principal source of vegetables and fruits in Parramatta's local market into the 21st century.[44]

The 1850s gold rush was the next event to significantly impact Parramatta's food supply. The fleet of passenger ships that delivered the influx of immigrants heading to the "gold diggings" was followed by shipments of goods to supply the increased demand of a growing population. Diggers travelling to and from the goldfields passed through Parramatta. While travellers heading to the goldfields required basic food supplies, returning diggers with their new-found wealth wanted a better quality of foods and even exotic high-status foods, such as French preserves, truffles and pâté de foie gras, that were supplied from Sydney wholesale importers on the newly completed railway service (1855).[45] With the end of the gold rush in the 1880s, many Chinese gold-rush immigrants who remained established market gardens and provided a more diverse supply of produce to the marketplaces.

Australian dietary patterns primarily have their roots in 18th- and 19th-century European cuisine and, in particular, the dietary patterns of the British Isles. The 1820s brought increasing varieties of imported foods. Factors influencing this transition were the improvements in the mechanisation of preserving techniques, marketing and transportation; in Britain, commercially preserved foods did not reach the market until the 1830s due to their high price. However, these technological factors eventually influenced the Australian market and gradually affected colonial dietary patterns.

---

36 Karskens 2010, 169.
37 Karskens 2010, 75.
38 Jervis 1963, 74–80; Karskens 2010, 83–97; Kass, Liston and McClymont 1996, 16–18; Tench 1793a, 55.
39 Clements 1986, 31.
40 Clements 1986, 32.
41 Karskens 2010, 151.
42 Barker 2015.
43 Artefact Heritage 2019, 78.

44 James 2010, 14.
45 Harris 2013, 37; *Sydney Morning Herald* 17 October 1859, 7.

6 The history of colonial medicine, public health and environmental reform

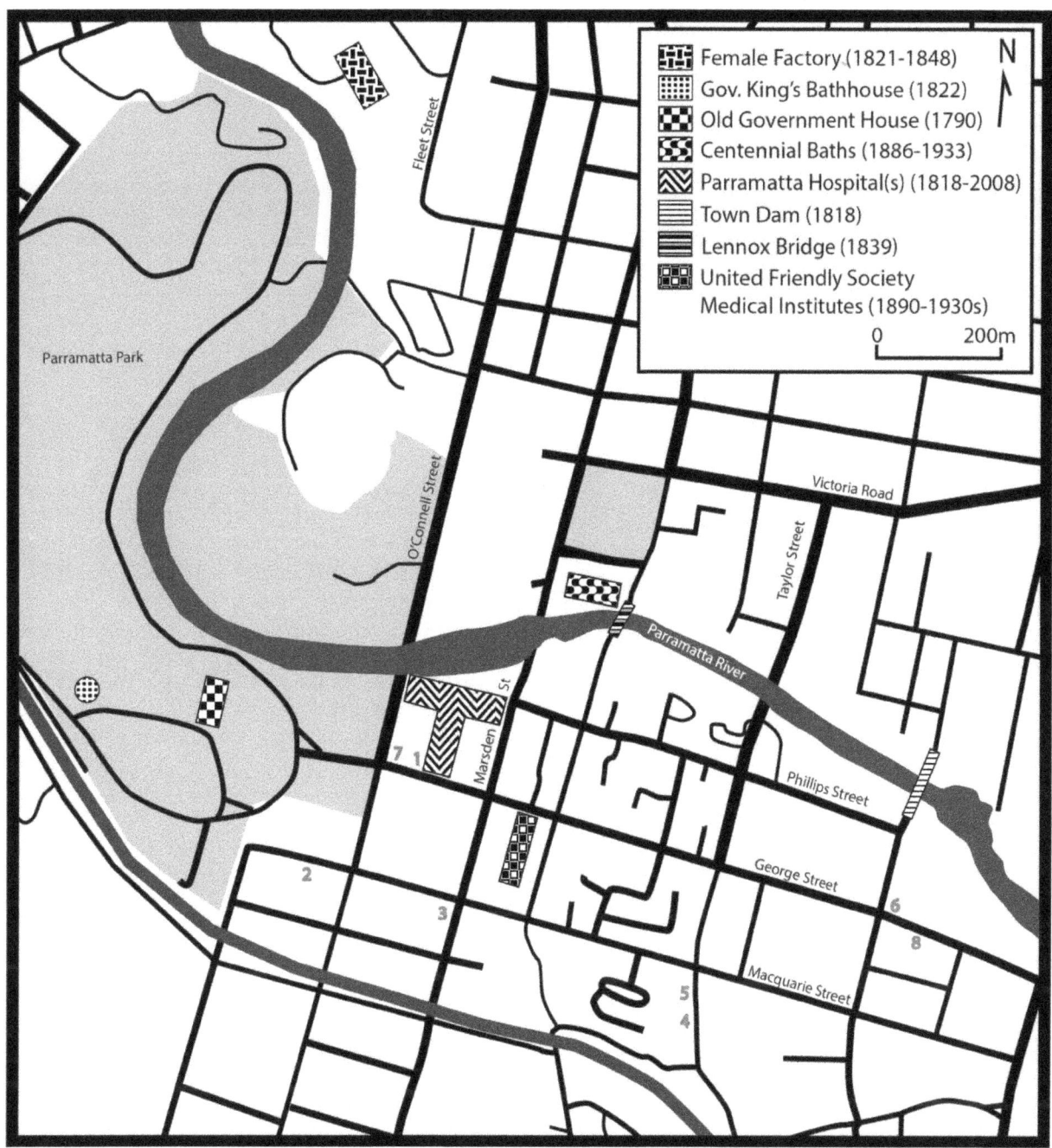

Figure 6.3 Plan Map showing Parramatta's structures that were institutions of health. Source: E.J. Harris 2021.

Institutions of health

In 1790, the first colonial hospital built in Parramatta was a temporary tent structure with a 200-bed capacity. This capacity might seem excessive for a population of 600 men, women and children. Nevertheless, Captain Tench, who was in charge of the newly settled outpost at Rose Hill, observed that on one day alone, the sick list contained the names of 382 persons.[46] The second hospital, built in 1792, was a permanent structure made of locally sourced bricks. It also had a 200-bed capacity. The hospital rapidly deteriorated and was replaced in 1815 by the Colonial Hospital, a two-storey brick structure that housed 100 patients. In 1821, the Parramatta Female Factory opened (Figure 6.3). This institution included a lying-in hospital to provide maternity and delivery care to the female convicts housed within. It also extended its services to non-convict mothers; however, records for the Female Factory indicate that only ex-convict women used this service.[47] With the closure of the Female Factory in 1848, obstetric services were sought at the Colonial Hospital.

---

46 K.M. Brown 1937, 2.

47 Reese 1991, 157.

As the population grew over the next 80 years, much-needed expansions to the Colonial Hospital resulted in a complex of structures to house and serve patients, including a kitchen, a laundry, an operating theatre and a separate ward (hospital) for the insane, which also served as an isolation ward for contagious diseases.

During the early settlement of Parramatta, the hospital was the only such facility where convicts and non-convict paupers could be treated. Yet, many of these disadvantaged non-convict settlers refused to seek treatment from this facility because it meant associating with convicts in open wards.[48] This attitude prevailed until the Parramatta Benevolent Society took over management of the hospital in 1848 and instituted segregated wards. Unfortunately, this segregation did not extend to the isolation of contagious patients, such as those with tuberculosis, until the 1880s.

Friendly societies

A friendly society (sometimes called a mutual society, fraternal organisation or rotating savings and credit organisation) is one of Australia's earliest manifestations of activist civil society. Unlike benevolent or charitable organisations, a friendly society is a collection of private individuals seeking solutions to collective, as well as to individual, problems. Australian mutual associations, among other goals, offered members affordable funerals, insurance, pensions, medicine discounts and cooperative banking. Pressured by both mutualists and the elite, the Victorian middle class in Britain accepted friendly societies as respectable organisations. By the mid-19th century, the societies had reached such levels of respectability as to achieve freedom from middle-class supervision.[49]

Australian friendly societies were initially comprised of commonplace people – tradesmen – who came together to pool their scanty resources to obtain some basic medical and other essential services they lacked. The first friendly society in Australia was established in 1830 in New South Wales, and the establishment of societies in other colonies soon followed. Within a few years, each colony enacted friendly society legislation, and by the 1860s friendly societies were a major part of life in every Australian town. As they evolved, Australian friendly societies came to have a much wider membership. While the cost of membership excluded poorer sections of the working class, by the late-19th century the membership of the leading national institution – the Australian Natives' Association – encompassed membership that ranged from professional men to labourers.[50]

Australia had no poor laws – laws that placed able-bodied poor in workhouses in Britain. Australians regarded the poor laws as a symbol of what they wanted to escape from the old world. Ratepayers, who would be required to pay a poor rate to support such laws, believed there should be opportunity for all in Australia and no need for poor laws. The reliance on benevolent (charitable) societies, like the Parramatta Benevolent Society formed in 1838, became the Australian path for assistance for the misfortunate – the aged, invalid poor, homeless children, unemployable and deserted wives. But the strain on charitable resources meant that they were not sufficient to meet the needs of these unfortunate people. Therefore, the inadequate funds of charities were supplemented by government money, raised not by land tax, but by selling off government capital assets and import taxes. The closest facilities to a British workhouse were public hospitals and asylums, in which the health care of the aged and the infirm poor was attended to.[51]

Throughout the 19th century, 10 per cent of Australia's population lived in a state of poverty,[52] yet the Australian middle class came to believe that Australia was "the working man's paradise".[53] The middle class found the possibility of poverty in this land of plenty incomprehensible, and, by the late 19th century, a middle-class movement led to official enquiries in all colonies into the charitable institutions and friendly societies to determine if, indeed, such services were needed.[54] In 1841 the Loyal Fountain of Friendship, an Oddfellows lodge, was Parramatta's first friendly society. During the next 45 years, no less than six other friendly societies were founded in Parramatta.[55]

Originally, Australian friendly society members joined to procure affordable medical care at prices they could afford. Each lodge or branch would have an elected medical officer to help assess sick pay claims, examine candidates for lodge membership and provide medical care, and often medicine, for each member who paid them an annual fee.[56] While there was a need for such a working-class organisation, few skilled or semiskilled workers took up the cover offered.[57] Instead, the cover was taken up by the unskilled working class. The societies' medical officers also had private practices, and some of these doctors began to view friendly societies with hostility. The issues were that their association with these mutualist organisations caused a loss of social and professional standing; poor performance led to the reduction of their payment as punishment; and the private practices were angered by participation in the medical schemes by men who could readily afford full fees as a private patient. For their part, the societies became concerned over the preference of part-time medical officers to focus more on their private practice and used the institute as a place of recruitment for their private practice.[58] In response to

---

48 R. Campbell 1983, 39.
49 Cordery 1995.
50 Hirst 2009, 141.

51 Hirst 2009, 127–8.
52 Roe 1975, 130.
53 Kingsley 1860, 994.
54 Evans 1983, 204.
55 Jervis 1963, 127.
56 Green and Cromwell 1984, 76.
57 Evans 1983, 203.
58 Hirst 2009, 96.

6 The history of colonial medicine, public health and environmental reform

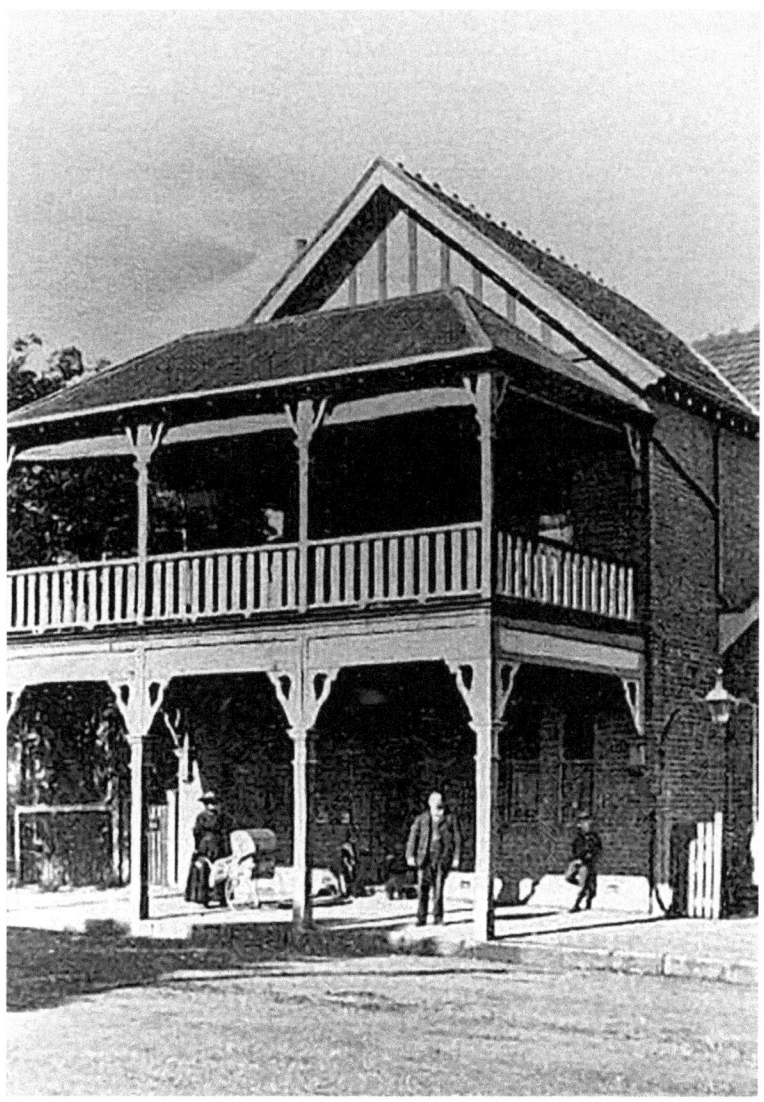

Figure 6.4 A c.1908 view of George Street showing the Parramatta United Friendly Society Medical Institute. Source: City of Parramatta Research and Collections.

this increased concern on the part of the societies, lodges began to join together to raise funds to establish and run a medical institute that would employ full-time salaried medical officers.[59]

The first medical institute established in Australia, and in fact in the world, was founded in Sydney in 1847 by Manchester Unity. The Parramatta and District United Friendly Societies' Medical and Dispensing Institute was established in 1890 (Figure 6.4). The institute was formed by the cooperation of 11 local friendly societies, with the five largest being the Acorn United Ancient Order of Druids, Pride of Australia Ancient Order of Foresters, Loyal Fountain of Friendship Manchester United, Independent Order of Oddfellows and Saint Patrick Australian Holy Catholic Guild of St Mary and St Joseph.[60] By the early 1890s, the institute had two attending medical officers; it had expanded to include 15 lodges with 1,300 members, and, including dependants, there were nearly 5,800 potential patients, or roughly half the district's total population.[61] The institute's membership grew slowly over the next 20 years. One 1913 advertisement for a medical officer reported a membership of 1,500 with one medical colleague on staff.[62]

Beyond attending to the medical needs of Parramatta's membership, Parramatta's friendly societies also promoted good health through sponsored sporting activities, such as sports gatherings that included races for a variety of sports, including foot racing, bicycle and wheelbarrow races, and even a "single ladies" race. Not only did these events serve to promote good health through competitive physical activity, but they also served as fundraisers to build a friendly societies hall at Parramatta.[63]

---

59 Green and Cromwell 1984, 96.
60 Kass, Liston and McClymont 1996, 235.
61 Green and Cromwell 1984, 97–8.
62 *Sydney Morning Herald* 19 July 1913, 30.
63 *Sydney Morning Herald* 27 January 1894, 4.

Table 6.3 Dates identified for the development of vaccines for contagions.

Contagion	Date of vaccine development	Developer
Smallpox (*variola*)	1804	Edward Jenner
Cholera (*Vibrio cholerae*)	1885	Jaime Ferrán
Typhoid (*Salmonella enterica*)	1896	Almroth Edward Wright
Diphtheria (*Corynebacterium diphtheriae*)	1913	Emil von Behring
Tuberculosis (*Mycobacterium tuberculosis*)	1921	Albert Calmette and Camille Guérin

Management of diseases and epidemics

Throughout the centuries, many explanations for the transmission of infectious contagions have been theorised, including superstition and geographic and meteorological conditions.[64] The most prominent scientific theory, known as the miasma theory, was developed out of fifth-century BC Hippocratic teachings. This theory held that disease was caused by a noxious form of bad air that resulted from vapours emanating from rotting organic matter, and a person could become infected when vapours entered the body and distressed its vital functions.[65] Miasma was believed to cause diseases such as cholera, chlamydia and the black death (plague). The first major shift in evidence-based medical theories came during the mid-19th century when Louis Pasteur demonstrated that microorganisms are everywhere, even in the air. Pasteur's revolutionary breakthrough was the basis of "germ theory", which states that these pathogens can lead to disease.

Issues associated with people living in proximity to one another include communicable diseases and epidemics. For disease and epidemics, the emphasis here is not on the politics of 19th-century Australia. However, one cannot exclude the political role played by the regulatory agencies in the development of guidelines for reform that affected the population's health.

Isolation and immunisation are the primary proactive methods of combating a contagious disease. The threat of epidemic disease was a strong motivator for legislation governing quarantine and vaccination; not all reforms were readily embraced by colonists. Smallpox was the first contagion in colonial New South Wales for which a vaccine was developed (Table 6.3). While smallpox existed throughout Europe, Asia, and Africa since the tenth century, it remained a comparatively mild contagion until a virulent type of the disease became an epidemic in late 18th-century Europe.[66] The 1804 call for inoculation of the children of military personnel against smallpox was met with widespread resistance in New South Wales. This resistance prompted an open letter written by the colony's Principal Surgeon, Thomas Jamison, in which he attempted to calm the population by stating that cases of smallpox had been identified in the colonial population and encouraging the military staff to inoculate their children against the disease as a precaution in the event it arrived on Australian shores.[67]

A cholera vaccine was not developed until 1885, so to counter the possible infiltration of Europe's 1830s cholera epidemic, new environmental laws were enacted in Great Britain and its colonial outposts. In Australia, a new regulation for establishing permanent maritime quarantine stations by 1804 was enacted, to isolate potentially infected passengers arriving on its shores.[68] Inspection for evidence of epidemic disease among arriving maritime passengers was common practice for all convict ships. At first, the ships were quarantined in the harbour until the medical corps officers could conduct an inspection. By 1814, passengers were allowed to disembark under guard and inspections were conducted at temporary stations. Eventually, 12 stations were established at ports around the entire continent. The maritime quarantine station at Port Jackson (Sydney), established in 1828, was one of these first permanent stations. The station operated for more than 150 years (1820–1984), and during that time, 580 vessels and 13,000 passengers were quarantined.[69] By the late 19th century, the Port Jackson station was also used for quarantine during smallpox epidemics (1881 and 1913) and the 1900 plague.

The Port Jackson station's primary function was to quarantine passengers and crew arriving on overseas ships. There were also a few instances of the quarantine of colonial residents. The only record of the station's association with Parramatta was during the 1859 scarlatina epidemic when the 12th Regiment, stationed at Parramatta, was given permission to quarantine at the facility.[70]

Tuberculosis was another serious contagious disease in New South Wales. An ancient disease, the rise in cases of tuberculosis was linked with the urbanisation of European cities during the Industrial Revolution and the increased size of their slums. As medical historians propose, the spread of the disease to British colonies resulted from Britain's emigration policy that emptied

---

64 Karamanou, Panayiotakopoulos et al. 2012, 58.
65 Karamanou, Panayiotakopoulos et al. 2012, 58.
66 Cartwright 1972, 121.
67 Harris 2021, 188; Jamison 1804, 2.
68 Foley 1995, 17.
69 Foley 1995, 10–11.
70 Foley 1995, 67.

its slums, dispersing the occupants to settlements around the globe.[71] They further contend that this emigration policy was the reason that the peak for tuberculosis-related deaths in Britain was the 1840s, while the death rate in Australia peaked in the 1880s.[72] The stigma of tuberculosis as a poor person's disease is not without reason. Poor nutrition that weakened the immune systems and a cramped, unclean living environment served to spread the disease.[73]

In Parramatta, tuberculosis was present from the early settlement years. Affected patients were treated in Parramatta's second hospital (1818), but they were bedded in a general ward.[74] It is unclear when a separate ward was established to isolate these patients. By the 1880s, a separate tuberculosis ward to house patients was located in a designated building north of the Parramatta Hospital for the Insane (1878–1916).[75] Both of these facilities have been subject to archaeological investigations. Since tuberculosis patients at the second hospital were housed with the general patient population, no artefactual distinction could be made.[76] Only limited archaeological testing at the Parramatta Hospital for the Insane has been conducted resulting in evidence of a mill race, which is unrelated to the hospital itself.[77]

A key factor in the decline of contagious diseases was the acceptance of germ theory, which in turn increased awareness of the need for better professional and personal hygiene practices. Acceptance of germ theory led to improvements in medical practice hygiene and was also instrumental in the introduction of antiseptic surgery. In 1867, Parramatta surgeon George Pringle conducted the first antiseptic surgery in Australia.[78] The 1860s introduction of household disinfecting agents decreased germs' spread for everything from the common cold to serious contagious diseases.

Environmental reforms: multiple lines of evidence

Collectively, the interpretation of in situ archaeological remains, artefact analysis and environmental factors contribute significant insights into the evolution of Parramatta's urban landscape. Delineating the occupational layers and features in the stratigraphic deposits of individual sites furthers the understanding of how the city addressed its public health issues. The statistics provided by artefacts are twofold. Firstly, dated artefact deposits establish a date range for delineated features associated with drainage, water supply and sewerage initiatives – both public and private. Secondly, they contribute to the study of health issues confronted by residents living in adverse conditions. An understanding of environmental conditions encountered by settlers increases understanding of the need for public health initiatives.

The historical records chronicle facts regarding infrastructure initiatives that, in part, were designed to improve public health, mostly on a district-wide basis. Sources, such as the *Historical Records of Australia,* detail the government's steps to address these issues for the colony at large. The *New South Wales Government Gazette* reported proposals and outcomes of improvement schemes. Newspapers reported the public outcry for improvements. Yet, none of these records reflects individual circumstances and how residential location and social status affected people's independent efforts to cope with or change these adverse conditions. Excavation results for historic sites across Parramatta have the potential to contribute information that cannot be obtained from the written record.

Environmental reforms to improve community wellbeing are divided into two categories. The first category includes factors related to the physical environment itself, such as drainage, sewerage and clean water supply. The second category includes issues related to people living in close proximity to one another, such as communicable diseases and epidemics discussed above.

Until the early 19th century, the physical aspect of environmental health in colonial New South Wales received little government attention. Economic and technological advancements were achieved at the expense of community and workers' health. Residents were left to their own devices to combat environmental conditions that affected their wellbeing and livelihood. Increased urbanisation and industrialisation in the growing colony brought increases in environmental and occupational hazards. Finally, it became the onus of the government to take drastic measures to improve aspects of Parramatta's infrastructure that adversely affected its inhabitants' public health. The time had arrived when the need for public health initiatives outweighed the infringement on the personal rights of the individual.

To understand the adverse environmental conditions that confronted Parramatta residents during the 19th century and the resulting environmental reforms first requires an assessment of Parramatta's geographic setting and its climate, town layout and the nature of the built architecture. Located at the head of navigation on the Parramatta River, the historic site of Parramatta was established in a shallow riverine valley defined by low rolling hills to the north and south (Figure 2.2). The Parramatta River is formed by the confluence of two fresh water creeks (Toongabbie and Darling Mills creeks) 1,600 metres upstream from the tidal estuary at the original landing place for the settlement, which is now known as Charles Street Wharf. The settlement's location was selected for its proximity to a vast acreage of arable land and its accessibility to Sydney. Site selection did not

---

71 Carpenter 2010, 223.
72 Lewis 2003, 224.
73 Carpenter 2010, 224.
74 Cameron 2015.
75 Longhurst 2011, 148
76 Casey & Lowe 2005b.
77 Casey & Lowe 2018, iv.
78 Hagger 1979, 165.

take into account the hindrances resulting from the low-lying landscape.

A detailed study of the geology and topography of the town was conducted as part of Higginbotham's 1981 archaeological excavations of an early brick drain.[79] Despite the modern modifications to the landscape, the study determined that the entire town area sits on sandstone and shale bedrock with overlaying deposits of red clay subsoil and a clay loam topsoil, with a thin band of light grey clay in between. Along the river is a riverine terrace with an elevation of 8 metres or less. At the time of early settlement, this area was mostly used for industrial and commercial activities. Much of the town was laid out on a terrace with an elevation that ranged from 8 to 12 metres, with a later expansion on 12 metres of higher ground to the south. The topography within this terrace was undulating and consisted of a series of gullies and creeks.

Settlement of Parramatta commenced in November 1788. The first erected structures consisted of a redoubt, barracks, stores and other necessary buildings, which were located on the ascent of a hill with a creek to the east for freshwater supply.[80] Two tracks were cut across the site; one an east–west track that later became High Street (George Street), which ran parallel to the river, that was bisected by a track that ran south from the redoubt to a nearby bridge (Pitt Street).[81] These tracks formed the backbone for the 1790 official town plan. The need for an official town plan was recognised by Governor Phillip; the plan was drawn up by Augustus Alt and laid out by surveyor William Dawes. It employed a basic Baroque scheme – a scheme that was designed to put people in their place utilising a hierarchy of space and separation of the classes. It consisted of a systematic grid laid out between two set command points – the landing place and military barracks at the eastern end, and the redoubt and later Government House at the western limit of the grid, a distance of approximately one mile; High Street was envisioned as the town's grand avenue.[82] Implementing the infrastructure for this plan was not without difficulty. During Captain Watkin Tench's 1791 visit to Parramatta, he noted that to construct the "great" road from the landing place to Government House, many gullies had been filled in with tree trunks covered with earth.[83]

A grasp of the early architecture is the next step in understanding adverse environmental issues confronting early settlers. There was no one skilled with the organisation and integration of building techniques: that is, no architect. Building construction was accomplished by tradesmen, mostly carpenters, masons and brickmakers, who had received their training in England. The high humidity and ignorance of native natural materials resulted in a series of trial-and-error construction projects that more times than not ended with the collapse or quick decay of buildings. The first barracks and huts alike were constructed with vertical posts placed directly into the ground. At first, walls were framed up with studs filled in with woven wattle-and-daub. All exteriors were plastered with pipeclay. When the first winter rains arrived, the clay washed away, and walls collapsed.[84]

By 1790, many public buildings were rebuilt, including a stone barracks, a brick storehouse and the governor's one-storey house of lath and plaster.[85] This first Government House in Parramatta was Georgian style, but not much larger than a convict hut (44 feet by 16 feet), consisting of a living room, a bedroom on either side of a central hallway and a skillion at the rear. The building was extended in 1793 to include a two-storey outbuilding to the north and a single-storey addition to the south.[86]

Aside from the governor's house and military barracks, the first Parramatta dwellings consisted of 32 rudimentary convict huts erected mainly along the High Street (later George Street). According to a firsthand account by Tench (1790), these 25-foot by 12-foot single-storey huts were "built of wattles plastered with clay, and thatched". The reporting of thatch roofing may have been in error, for in 1788, Governor Phillip forbad the use of thatch on buildings with chimneys in the colony. The tiles at that time were low quality and not weatherproof, so instead, convicts were set to work making shingles from she-oak (*Casuarina*), which was found to split easily.[87]

The floor plan was very similar to the standard British vernacular rural cottages, consisting of two rooms with a fireplace and brick chimney in one of these rooms.[88] These timbers were similar to Sydney construction, however Sydney structures used timbers from the soft cabbage palm tree, where Parramatta structures used good hardwood timber sourced from the rolling hills around the settlement.

Chimney bricks were made of softer clay than those made at Sydney's Brickfield Hill. By the time construction began in Parramatta, builders had learnt through trial and error the necessity to use shell-tempered mortar instead of clay mortar to ensure the structural integrity of chimneys.[89] Good sources of limestone, located in the interior, were not accessible until the 1860s railway construction. Instead, female convicts were tasked with collecting shells, often from Aboriginal middens, along the beaches. The inclusion of a fireplace in every hut is more indicative of in-home food preparation than heating. Parramatta's climate is classified as warm and temperate with wintertime mean low temperatures of 6–8° Celsius.[90] The need for fireplaces for heating was minimal.

---

79 Lawrie 1981, 26–34.
80 Kass, Liston and McClymont 1996, 14–15.
81 Kass, Liston and McClymont 1996, 15.
82 Kass, Liston and McClymont 1996, 22; Miller 1988, 66; Parker 2006, 30.
83 Tench 1793b, 246.
84 Herman 1970, 4–7.
85 Tench 1793b, 195.
86 Kass, Liston and McClymont 1996, 26.
87 Cowan 1998, 16; Proudfoot 1988, 60.
88 Tench 1793b, 195.
89 Herman 1970, 15.
90 Australian Government Bureau of Meteorology n.d.

6 The history of colonial medicine, public health and environmental reform

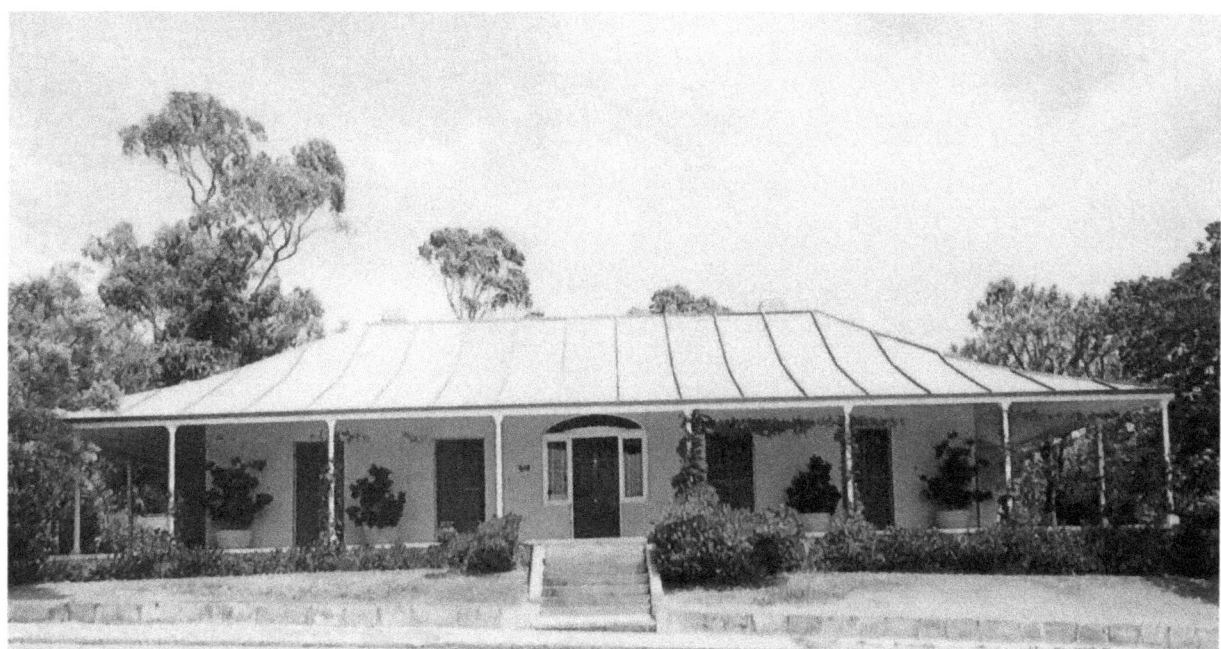

Figure 6.5 A 20th-century postcard showing Experiment Farm Cottage. Source: National Trust postcard: Ralph Cooke photographer.

No mention of flooring was noted in Tench's 1790 description of Parramatta. Parker's study of the construction of convict huts in Parramatta found that archaeological investigations produced no evidence of flooring. Yet, Herman's description of these huts states the floors and the fireplaces were brick and Higginbotham's excavation of a convict hut at 45 Macquarie Street located a brick floor (site 4).[91] Wattle-and-daub was used in the earlier Sydney huts, and its continued use for wall construction would contribute to the eventual deterioration of structures.

When Governor Hunter arrived in 1795, he wrote that buildings in Parramatta were in such a state of decay that they all needed to be repaired or rebuilt.[92] By the time emancipists began to lease town properties with huts in 1800, their condition had deteriorated, and many may have been abandoned. As the need for housing increased, Governor King ordered a major repair initiative, involving weatherboarding, whitewashing and "plaistering [sic]".[93] Parker's archaeological study of Parramatta convict huts indicates that significant repairs were undertaken on all huts, including replacement of vertical timbers for the rebuild of walls, lime-shell plaster to replace the previous clay daub, and the installation of glazed windows. Also, there is archaeological evidence that one or more of the huts had extensions.[94]

The first generation of buildings was never supposed to be anything more than temporary, providing a solution to the immediate need for security and shelter. In 1799 the simple governor's house was demolished and Governor Hunter commissioned the construction of what is now known as Old Government House. The first private home of any substance was a brick home at Elizabeth Farm, built in 1793 by John Macarthur. This structure was a simple, late 18th-century English vernacular cottage. Concessions to the colonial climate were made with the addition of verandahs to the house shortly after construction, inspired by the verandahs Major Grose had added to the Sydney barracks and Government House. With the addition of the verandahs, this four-room building (with hallway) evolved into what would become a model for the colonial homestead.[95]

There was no one architectural style in early Parramatta. John Harris built his cottage at Experiment Farm in about 1794, following an Indian bungalow's design, a verandahed style he observed in Bengal. Based on a traditional Indian design, this colonial Georgian rural dwelling responded well to New South Wales climatic conditions, maximising ventilation, shade and protection from heavy rain while meeting European expectations of form and comfort.[96] Conversely, when Rowland Hassall built his home in 1804, he built a two-storey classical Georgian cottage with quality bricks he had brought out as ballast from England. These permanent homes also demonstrate improved construction techniques, for Hassall's home stood for 78 years, and Harris' home still stands in the 21st century (Figures 6.5 and 6.6).

In 1823, as an incentive for improved construction, Governor Brisbane introduced a new form of lease for the

---

91 Herman 1970, 16; Higginbotham 1981; Parker 2006, 60.
92 Proudfoot 1988, 63.
93 *Return of Lands* 25 September 1800, 283.
94 Parker 2006, 60–7.

95 Historic Houses Trust of New South Wales 1995, 18–19.
96 New South Wales Office of Environment and Heritage, n.d.

Cleanliness is next to godliness

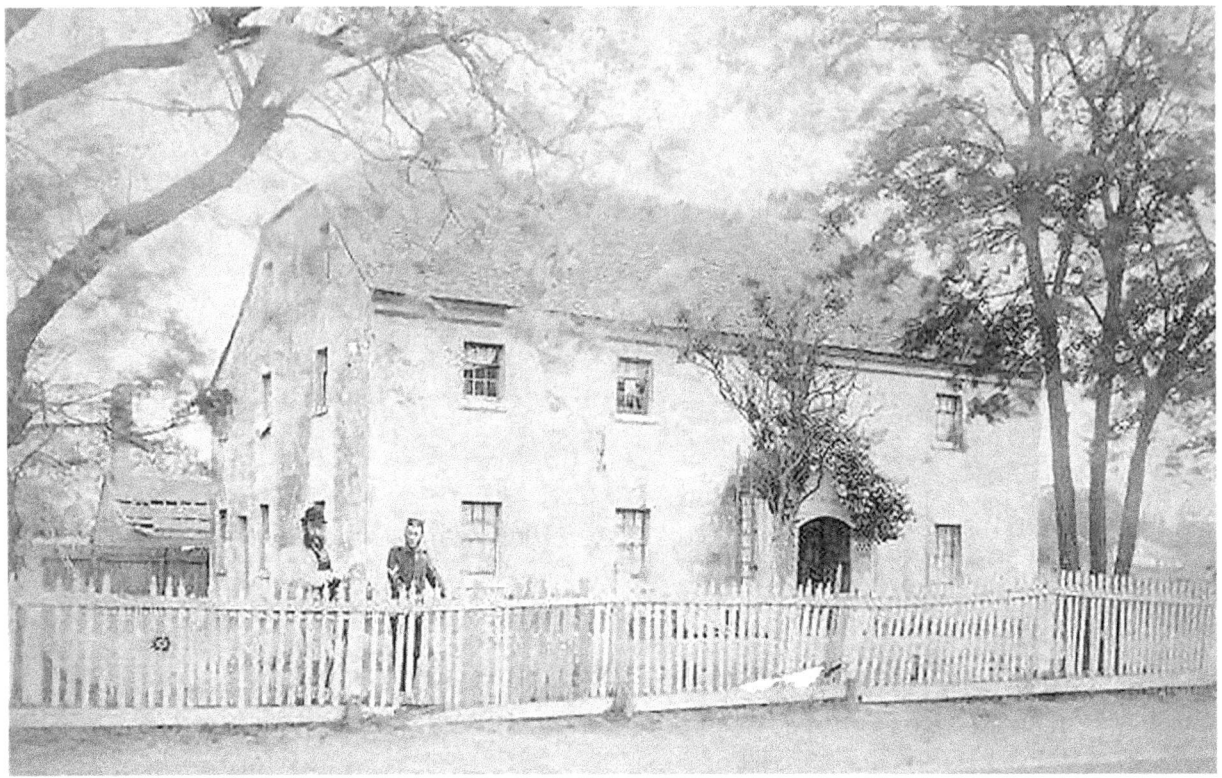

Figure 6.6 A photograph showing Aldine House, Rowland Hassall's home (1804–1882). Source: Courtesy of the Caroline Simpson Collection, Historic Houses Trust of New South Wales, Museum of Sydney (Historic Homes Trust: Record No. 42073).

town of Parramatta. It stipulated that 21-year leases could be obtained for 6 shillings quit-rent per annum. If the applicant had approved construction plans for a building costing at least £1,000, the lease would be converted to a land grant.[97] Of the 342 applications for leases in 1823, only 16 were converted to grants at the time of issue.[98]

As the number of converted land grants increased, so did the need to address increasing environmental issues that adversely affected the town. The calls for proper drainage, clean water and proper waste disposal are among the issues openly discussed and debated in printed media. Not only do these accounts detail the physical conditions that initiated the call for action, but they also describe the health issues associated with a population suffering from poor environmental conditions.

Like other colonial towns, there were many reasons for Parramatta's delayed response to sanitation issues, but apathy was not one of them. Public health initiatives were often undertaken in response to repeated public outcries for reform. The citizens of Parramatta were not silent when it came to voicing their calls for infrastructure schemes that would improve public health conditions. The public media of the day was the newspaper, and written calls for action, reports of public meetings and responses from council aldermen are commonly found in the archived regional newspapers.[99]

Throughout the 19th century, the most prominent infrastructure issues to affect the settlement's public health were proper drainage, fresh water and sewerage. The first issue to be contended with was drainage. Parramatta was chosen as the site for the second settlement based on its location on a fertile river crescent, and while the area was good for crops, the increasing settlement size and land clearing during the next two decades resulted in severe drainage issues. Poor drainage undermined the foundations of structures, and standing stormwater created health hazards, such as mould and mildew. Increased urbanisation also resulted in the pollution of the main water source, the Parramatta River. Industrial waste and sewage were major contributors to the pollution of the water supply; a sewerage scheme, therefore, became important to the wellbeing of the residents.

Among the citizens' calls to action was the 1863 call from residents for water-piping from the Hunts Creek Dam to Church Street, with moves for tenders set before Parramatta's municipal council.[100] Despite the continued public outcry from prominent residents such as Alderman Hugh Taylor (1865) and Dr George Pringle (1867), the town council continued to delay approval for

---

97 *Sydney Gazette and New South Wales Advertiser* 8 May 1823, 2.
98 Kass, Liston and McClymont 1996, 114.
99 *Sydney Morning Herald* 19 November 1867.
100 *Sydney Morning Herald* 4 February 1853, 8.

6 The history of colonial medicine, public health and environmental reform

the installation of a clean water supply.[101] An 1866 open letter published in the *Sydney Morning Herald* describes the Parramatta River's polluted waters and again calls for council to proceed with the proposed water-piping construction alongside an outline of their plan for such a system.[102] It also proposes the collection of the abundance of rainwater that falls on the town roofs for domestic use instead of letting it "run to waste".

Public and private health initiatives for resolution of Parramatta water issues

Information on Parramatta's public utility installations are detailed in two key volumes on water supply, sewerage and drainage in New South Wales and the greater Sydney area, both of which draw upon New South Wales colonial and municipal records to construct timelines for government initiatives.[103] Supplementary information on public health initiatives are public notices published in Sydney and Parramatta newspapers.[104] For the most part, these notices were calls for government action to improve sanitation, drainage and water supply in Parramatta.

During the early 19th century, no city in the world had a complete sewage disposal system.[105] In New South Wales, delays in the completion of sewerage schemes were often caused by political and financial factors. In Sydney, limited finance was the primary cause of a sewerage scheme not being commenced until 1854 when a New South Wales government loan backed it. Even when sewerage was completed in 1858, existing buildings were not obligated to connect to it, although all newly constructed buildings were required to.[106]

Government installation of sewerage and drainage infrastructure was a gradual process within Parramatta, in some cases spanning decades. The earliest public health initiative was the construction of brick barrel drains, which are historically referred to as "the convict drain" or "the town drain". Constructed in two phases (1820s and 1840s), it was a scheme designed to alleviate the boggy conditions in the low-lying areas of Parramatta Town. The surviving structure was first recorded in Higginbotham's 1981 archaeological investigations.[107] Subsequent archaeological excavations for the Parramatta Square redevelopment have identified other segments of this drain (Figure 6.7).[108]

Prior to the construction of the brick barrel drains, individual landowners struggled to deal with the boggy conditions. The low-lying property at 150 Marsden

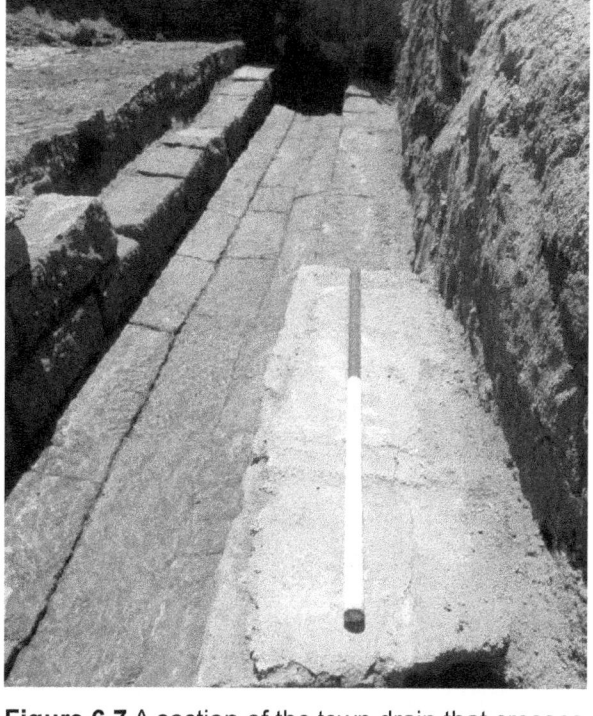

Figure 6.7 A section of the town drain that crosses 3 Parramatta Square. Source: Casey & Lowe 2016, cover.

Street (not a case-study site) represents one of the best examples of efforts of site build-up, where the ground level was raised and drainage systems installed to channel water away from homes and outbuildings. The property changed hands several times between 1810 and 1905, with each owner making efforts to improve the drainage system. Initially, small channel drains were excavated that emptied into a hand-dug sump pit. By 1820, a timber box drain was built on the downhill side of the house to draw the water away from the house. By the late 1800s, a French drain (a trench filled with gravel or rock, that redirects surface water and groundwater away from a structure or area) was constructed in the garden area of the property. Furthermore, layers of clay were laid down for at least four different building episodes to raise the ground surface.[109]

Figure 6.8 shows the elevations of sites in the case study and the course of the town drain. Archaeological evidence of efforts of landowners to control drainage is seen at sites in the case study where dams or ponds were constructed, and drains were dug in efforts to channel stormwater away from structures (Table 6.4). Results of archaeological investigations for case-study sites, described below, demonstrate the unique manners in which landowners attempted to solve drainage issues.

---

101 *Empire* 14 March 1865, 8; *Sydney Morning Herald* 19 November 1867, 3.
102 Harris 2021, 190.
103 Aird 1961; Henry 1939.
104 Harris 2021, 190.
105 Cowan 1998, 18.
106 Aird 1961, 128–9; Coward 1988, 89.
107 Higginbotham 1981.
108 Dusting 2016.

---

109 Kottaras 2009, 39.

53

Cleanliness is next to godliness

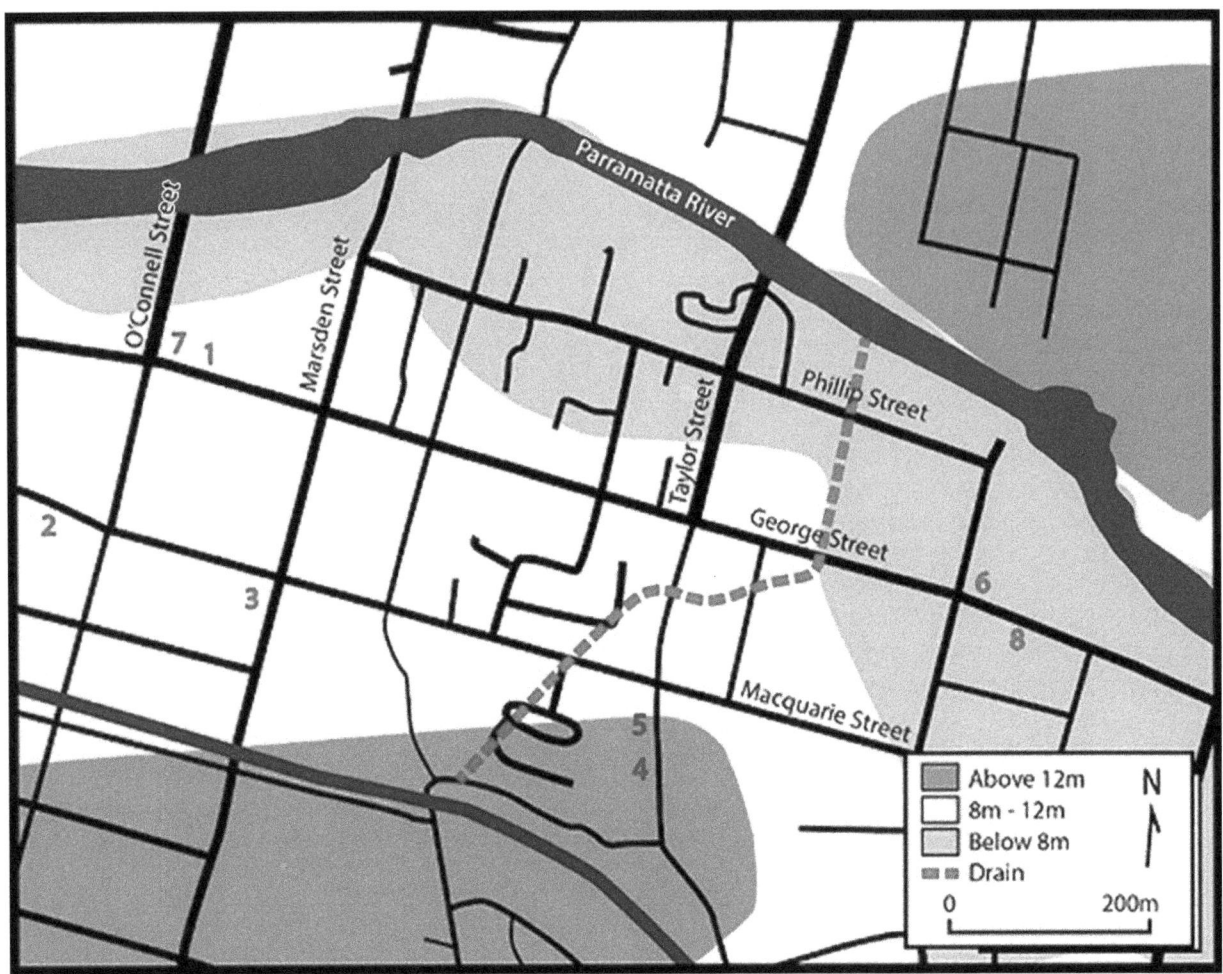

Figure 6.8 Plan map of Parramatta showing elevation and the course of the Town Drain. Source: based on Higginbotham 1983.

- **Site 2 – 15 Macquarie Street, Parramatta** A few blocks west of low-lying 150 Marsden Street was the property John Noble leased at 15 Macquarie Street in the 1820s. Located on an alluvial floodplain, the site was relatively level, gently sloping to the east where a creek ran north to the river.[110] This property had a natural pond that was expanded by hand excavation, creating a dam; two unlined drainage cuts leading to the dam were also dug. Like several other natural ponds in the nearby Domain (formerly Government Farm), it was used for drainage run-off. The dam was only filled in when improvements were made to the property, including a new stone structure in the 1840s, with a network of tile drains designed to channel stormwater run-off away from the structure.[111] The house at 15 Macquarie Street was built in the early 19th century (1800–1805) and stood until the 1850s when it was demolished. It was a rectangular shape and originally consisted of two rooms, one at the front and one at the back. It had a chimney at the rear. The house did not conform to the east–west alignment common to convict huts. The house was of timber construction and the narrow spacing of these timbers suggests the house may have had wattle-and-daub walls. Alteration to the property during the 1820s included additions to the north and west, which required additional drains to carry away the roof run-off.

- **Site 3 – 45 Macquarie Street, Parramatta** When John Walker acquired a 21-year lease for this property in 1823, a 1790s convict hut occupied the land. Leaving the hut as a workshop, Walker built a masonry home in 1836. This property was located on an alluvial floodplain, and had similar drainage problems to 15 Macquarie Street, despite the construction of an extensive drainage system to divert stormwater away from the modified convict hut that was standing on the property when Walker purchased his lease. The subsequent structural failures identified during the archaeological investigation probably resulted from the failure of these measures to adequately address the drainage issue, because the subsequent brick structure underwent substantial repairs for damage resulting

---
110 Casey & Lowe 2012, 65.
111 Casey & Lowe 2012, 12–13.

Table 6.4 Summary showing drainage issues for case-study sites.

Site number	Elevation (metres)	Drainage issues	Natural drainage	Soils description	Land formation	Archaeological evidence of constructed drainage
1	8–12	Yes	Creek	Sandy topsoil/subsoil	Alluvial slope	Drainage trench to creek; levelling fill
2	8–12	Yes	Ponds/creek	Sandy clay loam/hardset clay loam	Alluvial floodplain; gentle slope	Dam and unlined drainage channels
3	8–12	Yes		Sandy loam/clay	Alluvial floodplain	Series of drains and levelling fill episodes
4	> 12	No		Topsoil/clay	Hill slope	Stormwater drains
5	> 12	No		Clayey loam/silty clay	Hill slope	Stormwater drains
6	< 8	No	River	Topsoil/sand/bedrock	Alluvial slope	None
7	8–12	No	Creek	Sandy loam/clayey sand/sandy clay	Alluvial terrace	None
8	< 8	No	River	Sand/bedrock	Alluvial terrace	None

from stormwater. Also at that time, "a major lateral drain was cut across the slope a small distance behind the house, no doubt to protect the house from further stormwater damage".[112] By the 1880s, the front yard was raised with several episodes of levelling fill, which allowed stormwater to drain into the street.

- **Site 1 – 4 George Street** A convict hut was built on this property during the 1790s, and in 1837 James Harrex constructed a stone house on the allotment. Evidence of an early drainage trench at 4 George Street, located on an alluvial slope, was identified during archaeological excavations. This trench ran down towards an old creek line in the north-west corner of the property.[113] No subsequent drains or levelling fills were noted; as the naturally sandy soil at this property is much like that at nearby 2 George Street, no constructed drainage was required.
- **Site 7 – 2 George Street** When viticulturist Anthony Landrin arrived in Parramatta, he was provided with a convict hut at 2 George Street. In 1814 Samuel Larkin acquired the property, which, in an 1824 property dispute, was described as having a weatherboard house. In 1882, bookseller Cyrus Fuller built a new house on the site. While remnants of these three structures were found during archaeological excavation, no drainage systems were identified. The natural sand in the area allowed for quick draining of rainwater and a natural creek across the property appears to have been adequate drainage for the property.[114]

Other properties in the case study demonstrated only minimal need for constructed drainage systems.

- **Site 4 – 2 Taylor Street and Site 5 – 13–15 Taylor Street** The houses located along the west side of Taylor Street, between Macquarie and D'Arcy streets, were constructed in the 1870s. They were located at one of the higher elevations in historic Parramatta. While archaeological investigations of these sites did not record the natural soils, the high elevation and high slope gradient of these properties suggest that drainage was most likely never an issue. The only drainage systems encountered during excavation are stormwater drains that would have been connected by 1910 when the sewerage scheme was completed.
- **Sites 6 and 8 – 100 and 109 George Street** The structural remains of both the Byrnes home and the Hassall home were identified during archaeological excavations, but no evidence of drainage systems was located. The properties were located on a sandy alluvial terrace on the south bank of the Parramatta River. The sandy, silty soil provided adequate drainage for the properties.[115] Furthermore, the natural slope of this land to the river allowed for natural drainage.

As discussed above, in 2008, an analysis of pollen samples from 11 archaeological investigations in Parramatta

---

112 Edward Higginbotham & Associates 2007, 17–19.
113 Casey & Lowe 2005b, 6.
114 Casey & Lowe 2006b, 60.
115 Casey & Lowe 2006a, 48.

attempted to answer several research questions on topics such as agricultural and horticultural practices, colonial diet and environmental conditions. The study included three sites used in this case study (site 7, 2 George Street; site 6, 100 George Street; and site 8, 109 George Street). Results relating to damp conditions indicate that there was significant evidence of pollen and spores from ferns within or adjacent to drains for most sites in the town. These ferns occur naturally in damp gullies and on the margins of wet forest lands, suggesting significant damp issues alongside standing structures of most sites.[116] "Weed" flora found in pollen samples from site 7 is also indicative of damp conditions. Despite the proximity to the river, wetland taxa were not well-represented in the samples from sites 6 and 8.

Poor drainage resulted in standing stormwater; the resulting damp penetrated walls and floors, promoting mould growth that affected the health of the occupants of low-lying homes. Continued exposure to moulds often led to adverse medical allergic conditions, such as respiratory ailments and skin rashes.

Politics was the primary cause of construction delays to Parramatta's mid-19th century sewerage schemes. The Parramatta council declined to fund new drainage construction projects, contending that most of the drainage issues related to the numerous government institutions located in Parramatta and arguing that the New South Wales government rather than local ratepayers should pay for construction.[117] Under the 1905 *Parramatta Sewerage and Drainage Act*, the city-wide sewerage scheme was commenced; it was completed in 1910 with the government, on behalf of its various institutions, contributing £1200 for services rendered.[118]

The issue of rubbish dumping in public areas was addressed in Parramatta's 1897 *Municipalities Act* and included controls on the pollution of waterways, in the vicinity of the public wharf, and at the public market.[119] But it was not until 1904 that Parramatta council instituted new by-laws overseeing the municipal removal of household rubbish.[120]

The need for clean water supply in Parramatta

For early residents of Parramatta, sufficient access to clean drinking water was not a problem. Indeed, one of the reasons the site was selected for settlement was the accessibility of fresh water from the Parramatta River. Yet clean water supply became an issue within 20 years of settlement. Parramatta was the first settlement outside Sydney to contend with the issue of freshwater supply.[121] It was difficult to draw water for household use from the river. During early settlement, water for drinking, cooking, laundry, washing and bathing, and cleaning the house all had to be hauled in buckets from the river. In 1813, a public well was sunk in Macquarie Street; two years later another was sunk at an unidentified location in town.[122] In 1818 Governor Macquarie improved conditions by having a "town dam" constructed along the riverbank, which afforded easier access to the river's water supply.

Archaeological evidence suggests that by the 1820s some residents in the case study sought alternative sources of water by digging wells. It cannot be ascertained if these wells were a convenience or an attempt to procure a cleaner water supply. By the 1830s waterways were polluted due to overuse by an increased population and by government and private industries. Between 1791 and 1847, the population grew from 260 to 4,500 (Table 2.2) and an exponential increase of contamination in the water supply was inevitable.

In the 1850s the water demand necessitated the construction of a dam, and a site on Hunts Creek was selected; it would still be 20 years before the water in the dam was used. In the meantime, the council's water committee investigated its right to lay water and sewerage lines across private property. By the 1880s lines had been laid, but only 100 connections had been accomplished. It was not until the Sydney Water Commission took over management in the 1910s that efforts were made to connect every household and business.[123]

Water contamination

Contamination of Parramatta's primary freshwater source took many forms, with many resulting health issues. Use of the river for bathing and laundry were mild pollutants to the river, and, as the river became more polluted, these practices were abandoned. The alternative to river bathing was the Centennial Baths. Public baths were introduced in Britain in the 1840s. Robert Stanley of the Health of Towns Commission introduced a scheme that promoted national baths for the working class in cities such as Lambeth, Liverpool and London.[124] Following the model of Stanley's scheme, the construction and maintenance of the riverside Centennial Baths in Parramatta was made possible by the 1886 *Parramatta Public Baths Act*.[125]

Cattle and livestock were also a source of pollution. In an 1866 open letter to the habitants of Parramatta on the contamination of the river, one anonymous citizen comments that "the cattle from the Domain often take occasion during the summer evenings to walk in and very leisurely bathe themselves".[126]

A major source of contamination was drainage and raw sewage from the large government institutions such as the Industrial School for Girls, mental hospital,

---

116 MacPhail and Casey 2008.
117 Kass, Liston and McClymont 1996, 221.
118 Aird 1961, 161.
119 *New South Wales Government Gazette* 6 February 1899, 1096.
120 *Government Gazette of the State of New South Wales* 28 June 1904, 5093.
121 Larcombe 1973, 204.

122 Jervis 1963, 157.
123 Jervis 1963, 157.
124 Jackson 2014, 140.
125 Levine 1996, 1186.
126 *Sydney Morning Herald* 9 May 1866, 3.

George Street asylum, police barracks and gaol, which flowed into the Parramatta River as early as 1804.[127] One example noted during the archaeological excavations at Parramatta Hospital was a block of cesspits that included an overflow system that drained towards the river.[128]

As the population increased, pollution through drainage from private properties became a contributing factor to contamination of the Parramatta River. Residential properties close to creeks that fed into the river, such as 2 George Street, constructed systems for agricultural and stormwater drainage. Pollen analysis results of soil from drainage channels at 15 Macquarie Street suggest that the channels were also used as de facto latrines.[129] Wastewater containing raw sewage can carry parasites (tapeworms, threadworms and hookworms) and bacterial germs that cause diseases (salmonellosis, shigellosis, diarrhoea, trachoma and melioidosis) that can be transmitted to anyone who obtained their drinking water downriver of the discharge location of any such polluters.

Noxious trades

During the 18th and 19th centuries, flour mills, textile mills, breweries, distilleries, tanneries and wool scouring (wool washing) plants were major industries in Parramatta. The Royal Commission on Noxious Trades (1882), which investigated all manner of pollution into Australia's waterways and air, included these industries on its list of noxious trades.[130] These industries contributed organic or inorganic pollutants, or both, to the waterways. Pollution from these industries also contributed to airborne pollutants such as spores, ash and dust. Odours from these industries ranged from very unpleasant to noxious. The Royal Commission on Noxious Trades also highlighted abattoirs and slaughterhouses, butchers' premises, piggeries, meat preserving establishments, hide and skin store yards, boiling-down establishments, manure manufacturers, bone mills, breweries, distilleries, earth closet manure depots, tallow-chandlers, soap boilers, fellmongers, wool scourers, glue factories, tanneries, maizena and starch manufactories and paper mills as sources of pollution.

Flour mills were not listed as one of the 1872 Royal Commission's noxious trades, but they were contributors to the pollution of the waterways and air. Early water-powered flour mills, such as the one George Howell built in 1828 (Figure 6.9) and the 1840s riverfront steam-powered flour mills of Henry Harvey and the Byrnes brothers would have produced clouds of flour dust that caused respiratory ailments in workers and nearby residents.[131] While little was wasted during grain milling, any spillage of flour contaminated the water, making a foul-smelling paste that deoxygenated the water, killing fish and other waterborne organisms.

From early settlement, breweries were established all along the Parramatta River's banks. The first was James Squire's Malting Shovel in 1796, which was located at Kissing Point, on his 30-acre riverfront grant that was halfway between Sydney and Parramatta.[132] Within Parramatta, there were four breweries established during the 19th century, one of which was located on George Street on the south bank of the river. Established as the Burton Brewery in 1822, the business and property were subsequently purchased by William Byrnes in 1833; after the business closure in 1854, the property became an extension of the gardens of the Byrnes family home at 100 George Street.[133]

The brewers' waste was primarily mash that was traditionally used as animal feed. The only offences related to brewing the commission considered were the cleaning of casks and putrefied yeast, which caused an offensive odour when draining openly into waterways. Any such organic discharge also resulted in an increase in pollution through increased nutrient load, mainly nitrogen and phosphorus, but these were not noted in the commission's report.

Tanneries, textile mills and wool scouring industries located on the Parramatta River banks and its upstream tributaries were also serious contributors to the pollution of the river by adding too many nutrients into the water, effectively acting as a fertiliser that caused excess growth of algae. According to a study of late 19th-century European riverfront industries, textile and wool scouring industries were the major nutrient load polluters of the day.[134]

Due to the scarcity of imported leather in the colony, tanning was one of the colony's first industries. The tanning industry boomed quickly when native black wattle bark was used as an acceptable substitute for the English oak bark, a traditional source of tannins used to cure hides.[135] In 1821, Andrew Nash started his tannery on Phillip Street, which overlooked the river. Tanning is a tedious multi-step process and a great deal of water is required to wash and clean the animal hides. Removing the hair from a hide or skin required it to be soaked in a lime or water solution. To prepare a hide for tanning, it is steeped in a sour solution of rye or barley flour to raise the pores, making the hide more susceptible to the tanning process. The tanning process requires hides to be layered with crushed bark in a vat which is filled to the brim with water. Consequently, waste from tanneries consisted of a mix of inorganic and organic pollutants. Discharge of the spent solutions from the pits potentially contaminated two sources of drinking water: direct discharge into the river and leaching of tanning pits into the groundwater.

---

127 Aird 1961, 160.
128 Casey & Lowe 2005b.
129 Casey & Lowe 2013, 16.
130 Fitzgerald 2008.
131 Kass, Liston and McClymont 1966, 174.

132 Jones 2009, ix.
133 Jervis 1963, 105; Kass 2002, 9.
134 Billen, Garnier et al. 1999.
135 A.G. Brown and Ko 1997, 8.

Cleanliness is next to godliness

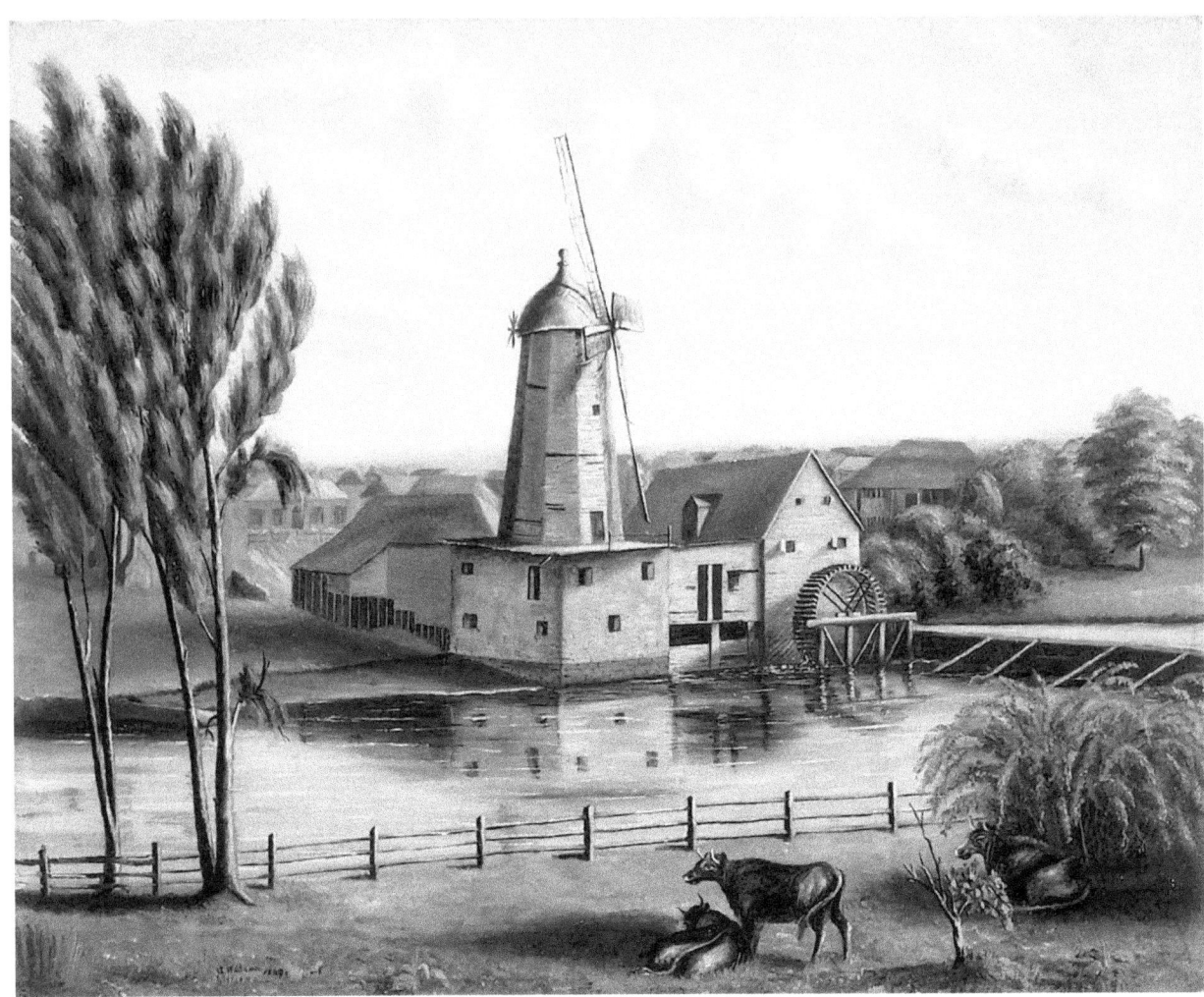

Figure 6.9 Howell's 1828 flour mill constructed on the banks of the Parramatta River. Source: State Library of New South Wales (a128324/ML 1050).

The 1882 Royal Commission on Noxious Trades contended with the disposal of both solid and fluid waste from tanneries. The commission found that little was wasted in the tanning process. Hair from the hides was either burnt or sold off for a binding medium used in plaster, and other animal by-products were boiled down and used as fertiliser. The commission did question the unrecorded nature and the amount of contaminated wastewater that was discharged into the river.

The commission was primarily concerned with the noxious smell of discharged fluids and recommended mixing fluids from the tanning pits with the lime-water solution (used in hair removal) before discharge.[136] While lime effectively neutralised the tannins, it did not completely dissolve the tiny particulates of organic matter suspended in the wastewater, which impacted the river water through the loss of dissolved oxygen. This loss was detrimental to aquatic organisms, which in turn promoted anaerobic activity that led to the release of noxious gases.[137]

Fortunately, there is archaeological evidence of the construction of the pits and their potential for leaching. Archaeological investigations of tanneries in nearby St Marys indicate that early to mid-19th-century tanning pits were often timber lined; by the late 19th century, pits were brick lined and later often cemented brick lined.[138] Potential leaching of solutions from the timber lined and uncemented brick-lined pits into the groundwater resulted in the contamination of drinking water in nearby streams and wells. Parramatta had several successful tanneries, including Charles Jackson's, which was established near the Hunter and Darling Mills creeks in 1847. Both waterways and the discharge from the tanneries eventually flowed into the Parramatta River.[139]

Similarly, the Byrnes brothers' facility for wool scouring and dyeing wool for weaving also used large quantities of water for processing. Upstream from

---

136 *Argus* 16 June 1871, 6.

137 Mwinyihija 2010, 22.
138 Green and Thorp 1987, 57–60.
139 Jervis 1963, 105.

6 The history of colonial medicine, public health and environmental reform

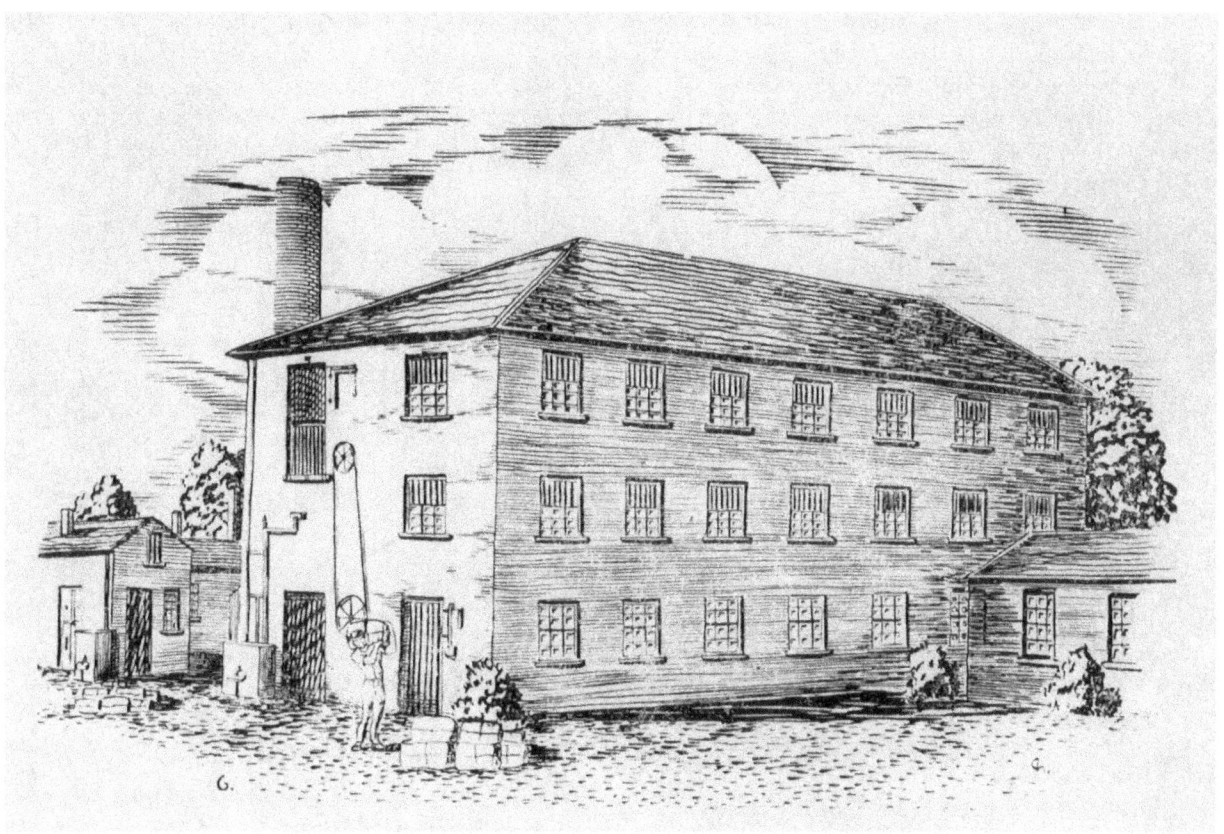

Figure 6.10 Sketch showing the 1841 Byrnes Steam Mill. Source: Rivett 1961.

Parramatta, near Toongabbie Creek, this facility was established after the mid-1840s expansion of the Byrnes brothers' George Street mill to establish a wool-weaving mill (Figure 6.10).[140] These two textile industries were significant contributors to the industrial pollution in Parramatta. Newly shorn wool is contaminated by impurities that need to be removed before the carding and spinning processes of yarn manufacture can commence. Impurities such as excrement, dirt and organic matter, and the natural suint (grease) in wool were removed in a process termed "wool scouring", which can reduce the wool (by weight) 40 per cent. Wool scouring is a process that washes the wool in a basket (often in a stream) before drying it in lofts or the sun. Once dry, rods are used to beat the wool to remove any remaining dust.[141]

The wastewater from tanning and wool scouring contained organic matter from cleaned hides and wool. Beyond the increased nutrient load in the waterways, the waste contributed to the threat of infectious disease. Anthrax first appeared in Australia in 1847 in Cumberland County, just south of Parramatta.[142] Tanning and wool scouring were the only industries to potentially spread anthrax through the discharge of what was later identified in 1876 as anthrax spore-bearing in waste into waterways where people bathed, swam and obtained their drinking water. Exposure to anthrax causes skin, lung and bowel disease in humans. Anthrax remained a severe health threat to livestock and humans until Louis Pasteur developed a vaccine in the 1870s.

Archaeological evidence of environmental reforms

Results of archaeological site investigations contribute to our knowledge of public health with the delineation of structural features, such as cisterns, privies, wells, water and wastewater pipes. Once municipal services were available to households, the cisterns, privies and wells were abandoned. Given the lack of municipal rubbish removal during the 19th century, the abandoned features were readily used for household rubbish. The historical record regarding the installation of services to individual addresses is sparse for Parramatta, and accounts such as Aird's 1961 volume *The Water Supply, Sewerage and Drainage of Sydney* are limited to dates for the starting and completion of such public health initiatives. Archaeological analysis of artefacts deposited in abandoned features serves as a further indication of when a feature was no longer serving its original purpose.

Similarly, the installation of municipal services also left temporal information in the archaeological record. The installation of underground water, drainage and sewerage pipes required the digging of a trench. The backfill of such trenches contains dated artefacts that

---
140 Kass, Liston and McClymont 1996, 174.
141 D.S. Taylor 2000, 267.
142 *Illustrated Sydney News* 5 December 1891, 9.

contribute temporal data regarding the installation date of these services.

There is archaeological evidence that each landowner in the case study attempted to resolve the problem of obtaining a clean water supply:

- Site 6, 100 George Street – a brick-lined well (context 3182) and a cistern (context 2207) were located on lot 70. Archaeological excavation of lot 70 found no evidence of structure associated with the Byrnes family (middle-class gentry), but rather a series of cesspits, a cistern and a well. A brick-lined well (context 2417) was located on lot 69, which is first noted on the 1895 plan of Parramatta.[143]
- Site 2, 15 Macquarie Street – the dam associated with John Noble's (working class) property may have been used as a domestic water supply or for livestock and agricultural purposes.
- Site 3, 45 Macquarie Street – the well at the rear of the John Walker and George Sweeney (middle class) property was lined with the same type of sandstock brick used in the construction of the 1830s masonry dwelling. This well was abandoned by the 1890s, as evidenced by the construction of an 1890s outbuilding over top of the well.
- Site 4, 2 Taylor Street – a brick beehive cistern was located at the rear of Henry Byrnes' property (middle class). It was constructed around the same time as the 1870s house built by George Coates.
- Site 5, 13–15 Taylor Street – a brick beehive cistern was located at the rear of the tenanted (middle-class) property. It was constructed around the same time as the 1870s semidetached dwelling built by George Coates.
- Site 8, 109 George Street – a pre-1830s well was located during archaeological excavation on the Hassall family property (middle-class gentry).

Efforts to obtain fresh water by sinking wells often failed. Bores sunk in low-lying locations often resulted in brackish water seeping into the wells.[144] This could be an explanation for the abandonment of the partially-excavated well at 4 George Street, and the early abandonment and the short timespan that the wells were in use at 100 and 109 George Street. The well at 45 Macquarie Street may have been abandoned after two major flooding episodes (1864 and 1888) destroyed the Macquarie Street dam across the Parramatta River. As early as the 1840s, carts were supplying water to households.[145] These carts may have supplied the cisterns at the rear of the Taylor Street properties. The cisterns could have been connected to piping to collect roof run-off, but no archaeological evidence of this was found.

In colonial Parramatta, public health improvement was related to various factors, including better nutrition, upgraded medicinal facilities and specialty health care for women. Benevolent organisations were formed to provide health care to the poor, and friendly societies were established to provide affordable health care to the working class. Environmental reforms, especially those concerning water supply, drainage and sewerage, were also important because of the increasing water supply contamination in the town.

This chapter uses archaeological evidence to show improvements to infrastructure, most notably drainage and installation of public services (water supply and sewerage) and historical evidence to show progress of government-operated medical facilities and government schemes for combating various disease epidemics. The next chapter describes personal healthcare options and seeks to identify the archaeological evidence in the artefact collections of the case study, in an attempt to identify influential healthcare patterns on a city-wide scale.

---

143 Miskella 2003a; b.
144 Jervis 1963, 157.
145 S. Brown and K. Brown 1995, 131–2.

Chapter 7
THE ARCHAEOLOGY OF PERSONAL HEALTH AND SOCIAL REFORMS

Ever present in the annals of Parramatta's history is a wealth of the public faces of its residents. In contrast, the archaeological records provide insight into their private lives. The marriage of these two disciplines provides a fuller picture of Parramatta's residents. One example of middle-class gentry is the Byrnes family. Historical documentation records that in 1853, William Byrnes built a Georgian manor as a home for his 11 children on seven contiguous allotments purchased on the north-east corner of George and Charles streets. William was a very successful businessman, a member of the Legislative Council, and one of the earliest members of the Freemasons. By the late 19th century, William shared his home with just his two spinster daughters, Emmeline and Marian, where he lived until his death in 1891.

Emmeline and Marian's public lives played out in the pages of the local newspapers. Emmeline's social outings were noted in several newspaper accounts, including articles on the Chemist Wholesalers' ball. While Emmeline was involved in religious and society activities, Marian Byrnes was also very socially active with civic and political matters.[1] As an officer of the Wesleyan Church's Women's Workers' Association, Marian organised a World War I knitting circle to provide socks and balaclavas to the troops, and was active in the War Chest Button campaign.[2] For several social occasions, her fashionable attire was noted in newspaper society columns.

A third Byrnes sister, Ann, married Dr George H. Pringle, but after his death, Ann resumed her place in the Byrnes household in 1921 along with her daughter Miss Alice Maud Hogarth Pringle. Young Miss Pringle, who lived in the family home until her death at the age of 86 in 1952, reminisced about the history of the family and the home at 100 George Street during a 1949 interview;[3] yet this history spoke little of the private lives of the family.

Some insight into the Byrnes' private lives is found in the analysis of the archaeological record. In a time of increasing Church-sponsored temperance activities, artefactual evidence demonstrates the extent to which the Byrnes household privately supported abstinence of alcohol and tobacco consumption. The affluent Byrnes family could afford professionally prescribed medications, but did they avail themselves of the increased popularity of patent medicine? What was their attitude towards personal hygiene? Did these hygiene practices carry over to their attention to household cleanliness? These are just a few of the questions addressed in the following artefact analyses.

Personal health relates to social reforms and the proactive and reactive approaches to wellbeing on an individual basis. Social reforms are considered within the theoretical framework of cultural interpretive approaches to the analysis of health and illness, but attention must also be given to both the occupied environment and the oversight of external political-economic influences.

Traditional medicine and self-medication

Home remedies are what might be termed in the 21st century "alternative" therapies or treatments, but in an extensive discussion of colonial Australian medicine in *Paradise of Quacks: an alternative history of medicine in Australia*, Philippa Martyr uses the term "alternative" for medicines or remedies that did not conform to orthodox medical practices of the time.[4] This astutely highlights that these alternative, or unorthodox, medicines were not the exception in 19th-century medical treatment, but the norm practised by most individuals.[5]

Many publications catering to this self-medication practice detailed the contents of a basic home medicine chest (Table 7.1).[6] Dinneford & Co., best known for their "pure fluid magnesia", sold medicine fitted out in medicine chests, much like those used by early colonial physicians, complete with a glossary of terms, explanation of medicines, recipes for compounding remedies and tables of doses, weights and measures.[7]

Some Parramatta residents may have taken advantage of homeopathic remedies obtained from trained physicians and chemists. Homeopathy is based on the idea of "let like be cured by like". Homeopathy became popular in the 19th century in part because of its success in treating epidemics.[8] Parramatta's first private-practice

---

1 *The Methodist* 15 March 1930, 20.
2 *Cumberland Argus and Fruitgrowers Advocate* 4 September 1897, 12.
3 *Cumberland Argus and Fruitgrowers Advocate* 26 October 1949, 1. See also *Sydney Morning Herald* 1 July 1952, 14.
4 Martyr 2002.
5 Martyr 2002, 268–72.
6 Beasley 1886.
7 Dinneford & Co. 1854.
8 Fisher 2012, 1.

Table 7.1 Basic contents found in a home medicine chest. Source: *Daily Mail* 26 June 2012.

Medicine	Description
Manna	A sweet substance obtained from various plants, especially from an ash tree, *Fraxinus ornus* ("manna" or "flowering ash"), used as a mild laxative.
Steers' opodeldoc	A liniment made from soap, spirit of wine, camphor, rosemary oil and sometimes spirit of ammonia.
Turkey rhubarb	A plant thought to have healing properties.
Peppermint water	Used to treat ailments such as diarrhoea, flatulence and vomiting.
Laudanum	Alcoholic herb preparation containing opium, which "seldom fails to occasion a calmness in the system whence its use in gout and spasmodic disorders".
Lavender	Herb used for digestive ailments, and "useful for cases of depression, sickness and languor".
Epsom salts	Used as a mild laxative and anti-inflammatory agent.
Cream of tartar	By-product of winemaking used as a laxative.
Double-distilled cardamon	An aromatic spice used for digestive relief.

physician William Sherwin (service 1829–40) was also the second homeopathic physician in New South Wales.

Traditionally, many people relied upon home remedies, consulting their home recipes that had been handed down from generation to generation. Some took their remedies from local newspapers that printed "tried-and-true" remedies as useful fillers for their readers' good, but often they were restricted by the potential loss of profit which they derived from the advertisements of makers of patent medicines.[9] Other people consulted one of the many published books, manuals and guides to treat ailments. Still, others turned to the highly advertised patent and proprietary medicines; many of them were available in Parramatta in the long 19th century. While traditional remedies leave no obvious evidence in the archaeological record, or even in pollen analysis studies, patent medicines leave behind their commercial packaging that can be subject to archaeological analysis. The author did a separate study exploring health concerns by analysing commercially packaged patent and proprietary medicines from a cross-section of colonial households.[10] This comparative study used eight archaeological assemblages from 19th-century Parramatta sites; six of these sites are included in this case study. The results of this patent medicine analysis are discussed below. Among the volumes written on the patent medicine phenomena, many explanations are given for the existence and rise in popularity of patent medicines; the most often noted include these:

- cost of professional medical care
- availability of professional medical care
- distrust of medical practitioners
- improved marketing and advertising techniques
- availability of and access to traditional medicine through "wise women"
- the Industrial Revolution, which caused a demographic shift from a predominately rural and agrarian population to a more urban population.

Physicians and medical practitioners

After home health care, an individual's next option was to consult available certified and uncertified medical practitioners, which consisted of an assortment of healers including surgeons, midwives, accoucheurs, barbers, bonesetters or empirics depending upon the health issue. The physician or surgeon was called upon for serious and life-threatening medical problems (Table 6.1).

As the population grew and the economy began to flourish, private medical practices began to spring up across the colony. At the beginning of the colonial period, physicians' treatments were extremely rudimentary and largely directed at the symptoms rather than the causes of infectious diseases. Dennis Considen, a surgeon on the First Fleet, was a colonial pioneer in developing remedies from native plants to treat dysentery, scurvy and other diseases.[11] Among these native plants were sarsaparilla and spinach, as well as oil of peppermint from eucalyptus trees and native myrtle that were astringents used to treat dysentery.[12]

For many major diseases confronting 19th-century society – consumption, diphtheria, typhoid, measles, pneumonia and heart disease – the physician had no established cures, nor did he fully understand the causes of these diseases. Fortunately, by the late 19th century, the germ theory of disease was finally proven and the germs that caused some of the worst contagious diseases were

---

9   Loomis 1949.
10 Harris 2019, 26–36.

11 Gilbert 1966.
12 Keneally 2006, 74.

identified, giving the physician new tools to eradicate and/or treat these diseases.

The 19th century saw significant medical advancements in the diagnosis and treatment of disease, as well as pain management, surgical techniques and preventative treatments (vaccinations):

- new drugs that were developed, including morphine, codeine, quinine and ephedrine[13]
- compulsory vaccination for smallpox was introduced in Britain in 1853[14]
- antiseptic techniques in surgery spread in the second half of the century[15]
- research by colonial surgeons at the end of the 19th century began to uncover the role of vectors, such as mosquitoes and ticks, in spreading diseases including elephantiasis and malaria, opening up the possibility of disease control through vector eradication[16]
- causal agents were discovered for typhoid, leprosy, malaria, tuberculosis, cholera, streptococcus, diphtheria, tetanus, plague and dysentery between 1880 and 1900[17]
- vaccines were developed for diphtheria, cholera, tuberculosis, tetanus, yellow fever and typhoid fever between 1890 and 1930.[18]

Of all the medical advances during the 19th century, the 1866 development of the portable clinical thermometer had the most profound significance and importance in diagnosing and treating illness by shortening the time to obtain a patient's temperature from 20 to 5 minutes. Its size (6 inches) made it a useful addition to the physician's medical bag when he was called to tend a patient away from his surgery.[19] To one physician's dismay, the science behind this new diagnostic medical tool eluded his patients, who believed it was the thermometer that was curing them.[20]

Newly discovered medicines had to be obtained from a qualified doctor – a rare individual in 19th-century Australia. Until medical schools were opened in in Melbourne (1862), Sydney (1883) and Adelaide (1885), all Australian doctors had to receive their training abroad. This period also saw a shift from alternative unregistered medical practitioners to a more regulated industry that was overseen by newly established governing medical boards (2 *Victoria, Act No. 22)*. While herbalists and bonesetters were still viewed as useful adjuncts to qualified medical practice, a series of new legislation was enacted over the 19th century to stop the practice of medicine by unqualified surgeons and physicians. The 1838 *Medical Profession Regulation Act* created the New South Wales Medical Board to determine whether applicants were qualified to be certified as medical practitioners. This Act also called for a list of qualified and registered medical practitioners to be annually published in the *New South Wales Government Gazette*. By 1900, the *Medical Practitioners (Amendment) Act 1900* (Act No. 33, 1900) was enacted to impose penalties on people using titles including surgeon or physician if they were not appropriately registered. Along with the increased regulation of medical practitioners came a shift in attitudes towards personal health care. As medical historian and philosopher Michel Foucault explains, with the advent of modern clinical orthodox medicine in the early 19th century, patients gradually lost their individuality and, in the eyes of the physician, were reduced to an example of disease.[21]

Women's health

Women's health in the 19th century centred on childbirth. Therefore, the good health of women was paramount to the survival of the colony, for without procreation, the colony would not thrive. Health care for the colonial woman was the most challenging concern for the Colonial Medical Corps surgeons who provided the majority of medical services to all settlers in the early settlement years (1788–1820). For medical issues unique to the female anatomy, especially difficulties during childbirth, these British-trained physicians were ill equipped to treat their patients.

One of the earliest accounts of difficult childbirth in Parramatta concerns colonial surgeon John Savage, who in 1804 failed to attend a woman in the throes of a difficult delivery. The woman's husband sought out Savage, telling him that the midwife in attendance believed delivery required skilled assistance with instruments. Savage sent the husband home with instructions for the midwife to exercise her discretion as there were no such instruments in Parramatta. He then he proceeded to mount his horse and set off for Sydney to tend to his own business. Despite the efforts of the midwife, the patient died. Surgeon Savage was tried by court martial, found guilty, dismissed from government service and sent back to England.[22]

Prenatal infant mortality (miscarriage) and stillbirth were also issues in the early years of settlement. Archaeological evidence of infant mortality was found during the investigation at the Parramatta Hospital, where remains of three perinatal in utero skeletons were recovered from deposits dating from the 1790s to the early 1800s. Two perinates were buried in one grave in the south-west corner of the hospital grounds, and one was recovered from the fill of a nearby cellar dated to the first quarter of the 19th century. The authors of a dedicated article on these remains note: "The two individuals in

---

13 Bynum 1994, 74.
14 Carpenter 2010, 93.
15 Lewis 2014, 201.
16 Lewis 2014, 201.
17 Carpenter 2010, 11.
18 Dyke 2014, S33.
19 Pearce 2003.
20 Martyr 2002, 19.

---

21 Carpenter 2010, 2.
22 K.M. Brown 1937, 6–7.

the grave were buried according to traditional Christian method in terms of their orientation, but they were not placed in individual graves and they were not baptised and were therefore buried in unconsecrated ground".[23]

Throughout the 19th century, an expectant mother of any class with no apparent signs of complications typically did not consult a physician or midwife during her pregnancy.[24] Potter's research on 19th-century traditional midwives in Sydney and surrounding communities (Parramatta, Windsor and the Hawkesbury) is the first comprehensive study in Australia of these practitioners and their profession.[25] The fragmentation of available information on midwives, pregnancy, confinement and childbirth complicated her research. Despite the number of diaries and letters written by colonial women, changing 19th-century cultural attitudes towards these topics cast a veil over their discussion due to their private nature and the perceived delicacy of the subject.

Contraception and abortion are other taboo topics in the written record. Contraception was not a subject most colonial families contemplated, as they tried to produce a family unit large enough to succeed them. Nevertheless, for those who wanted to avoid pregnancy, there were only a few available preventative measures. Within a family, the most common birth control method was likely *coitus interruptus*. Condoms as a contraceptive method have been around for millennia. The 18th-century version was made of skin or intestines and often treated with lye or sulfur as a chemical deterrent to curb the alarming rise of syphilis. Charles Goodyear's development of his rubber vulcanisation process resulted in the production of more durable rubber condoms that were produced on a large scale by the 1860s.[26]

Abortion and infanticide were techniques of birth control in Australia. Abortions were often too costly for working-class women and single women who needed to avoid the consequences of pregnancy.[27] One of the archaeologically recovered perinates noted above was discarded in the rubbish fill of an abandoned cellar, suggesting that it may have belonged to an unwed mother (possibly a female convict) or was intentionally aborted. Abortion was commonly achieved by women, such as Hannah Green, by ingesting excessive amounts of remedies and patent medicines.[28]

For other female-related complaints, women commonly practised self-medication. By the mid-19th century, several publications were written to assist women in self-treatment for common feminine disorders, including *The Married Woman's Private Medical Companion* and *Female's Medical Guide*.[29] These references generally recommend changes in diet, exercise and herbal remedies to treat female conditions ranging from menses, menstrual ailments and morning sickness. By the late 19th century, the first medical practitioner to specialise in women's medicine in Australia was Ellen Curling, who set up her practice in Parramatta at 2 Taylor Street (Site 4) in 1878. The concept of a specialist for women's medicine, especially a female practitioner, was so novel that it was reported in the *Australian Medical Journal*.[30]

Consumer choice for self-medication

Self-medication was the first source of treatment. Traditionally, treatment of common ailments relied upon home remedies that were passed down through families or found in printed media. For the most part, the anachronistic use of these remedies leaves no trace in the archaeological record. Patent medicines are one of the most widely written about aspects of 19th-century medicine.

The patent medicine industry had its origins in early 18th-century Britain and refers to medications whose ingredients had been granted government protection. Many of these medicines were not "patented", but rather proprietary medicines. One of the earliest known "patented" medicines was a cough and cold remedy, Daffy's (Daffies) Elixir, developed in the mid-17th century.[31]

The terms "patent" and "proprietary" are commonly used to describe packaged drugs that can be obtained without a prescription. Patent is shortened from "letters of patent", which was an open endorsement from a monarch or government that granted the sole right to make, use or sell packaged drugs, while other commercially packaged over-the-counter drugs are termed "proprietary".[32] From the late 18th century, British-manufactured patent and proprietary medicines became increasingly popular throughout Britain. By the 19th century, hundreds of British patent medicines to treat dozens of ailment types were available in Australia through established wholesaling networks.

A primary reason for the prominence of patent medicines in archaeological scholarship is the substantial amount of information regarding them found in historical documentation and the archaeological record. These medicines were advertised to the public by a trading name and purported to be effective against minor disorders and symptoms. While the term "patent medicine" is often used to describe quack remedies sold throughout the 19th and 20th centuries, it is beyond the scope of this work to distinguish between quack remedies and those efficacious formulations developed and sold by legitimate professionals, such as pharmaceutical companies, chemists and physicians. Rather it discusses the various possibilities for the rise in popularity of

---

23 Donlon, Casey et al. 2008.
24 Carpenter 2010, 163.
25 Potter 2017.
26 Youssef 1993.
27 Bongiorno 2012, 70.
28 Sprenger 2012, 75.
29 Mauriceau 1855; Skinner 1849

30 1878, 339.
31 Homan 2006.
32 Sprenger 2012, 13.

patent medicines in the Australian colonies and to a larger extent, worldwide.

Patent medicines are mentioned by name in private journals left behind as personal records of people's lives, referenced in literature and historical accounts, and are the subject of reports and commissions conducted by governments and medical organisations. During the 19th century, patent medicines were one of the most widely advertised commodities as evidenced by extant advertising cards, handbills, newspaper notices, almanacs and organisational journals. Graham's research on 19th-century medicinal advertisements in Victoria's newspapers identified more than 800 individual products, which she quantified into 35 separate ailment categories.[33] Archaeologically, commercial containers used to dispense and distribute this type of medicine were durable glass, which has survived in the archaeological record. Most recognisable of these medicines are those packaged in containers with embossed or enamelled labelling. While medicines distributed by compounding chemists were often packaged in embossed-labelled containers, embossed labels are often limited to the name and sometimes the address of the chemist and do not identify the medicine contained within.

Parramatta study of patent medicines: archaeological evidence

The author's 2019 study on health concerns in Parramatta examined numerous types of commercially packaged medicines.[34] This study aimed to determine which ailments residents chose to treat through self-medication and, through a comparative analysis, distinguish self-medication patterns by socio-economic status. It included more than 1,500 medicine bottles from seven residential sites (738 bottles), the town's chemist shop (774 bottles) and the Parramatta Hospital's surgeon's quarters (9 bottles). Artefact collections from a chemist's shop and the surgeon's quarters were included in the 2019 study for comparative purposes. The seven sites utilised in the 2019 study included six in this research. One site was excluded from this case study because it failed to meet the site-selection criteria as its occupants could not be identified. A review of the 2019 study is appropriate here, as it contends with the social aspects of self-medication.

The study was limited to analysing glass medicine bottles due to their abundance and robust embossed labelling. The range of medicine types goes beyond just patent medicines and includes compounding chemist, patent and proprietary, prescription, Chinese herbal and medicinal alcohol (schnapps) bottles (Table 7.2). One shortcoming of the study is that it did not present data for patent medicine types in tabular form for each household, but rather summarised the data in text. The presence of such data may have helped future researchers to delineate patterns in patent-medicine.

The 2019 study presents a hypothetical medicine chest based on typical product types found in all residential assemblages. Table 7.3 shows the relative frequencies of all medical complaints treated by the product types. A comparative analysis using medicine chest product types was conducted for households from different socio-economic classes. The analysis found similarities among classes and a few differences between these classes.

As Table 7.3 shows, cure-alls, patent and proprietary medicines that were advertised to treat multiple ailments represented approximately 45 per cent of medicines (excluding schnapps). As the study notes, ingredients in cure-alls frequently included opiates or a high percentage of alcohol, or both. Schnapps (33 per cent), also categorised as a cure-all, was discussed separately because it could have an ambiguous status as either medicine or alcoholic beverage. Table 7.4 shows that schnapps bottles were recovered from all household assemblages. As discussed later in this chapter, the increased use of medicinal schnapps was due to shrewd marketing that took advantage of the temperance movement's growing prominence to persuade *respectable* women to use the product for its many restorative properties. The 2019 study attributes the increased popularity of cure-alls and schnapps due only in part to the increased influence of the temperance movement in the 19th century.

Patent medicines for respiratory ailments (coughs and colds) were common in working-class household medicine cabinets. Besides relieving symptoms of the common cold, cough remedies were used to alleviate the symptoms of allergies (pollen, food and moulds) and industry-related respiratory ailments, such as byssinosis, an occupational lung disease caused by exposure to cotton dust. Opiates were a common ingredient in cough remedies due to their cough-suppression properties.

Medicines for gastrointestinal ailments (constipation, parasites and indigestion) represent approximately 29 per cent of patent medicines, and every household had at least one brand of fluid magnesia in the medicine cabinet, along with castor oil and effervescing salts. Generally termed laxatives, these medicines were commonly used for relief from constipation. Other uses of these patent medicines were to expel intestinal parasites, but more often they were taken to restore balance to the "humours", disordered by constipation or indigestion. It was noted that one cause for constipation was opiate-based medicines (cure-alls and cough remedies) taken for a range of other ailments.[35]

A noticeable difference was identified for the middle-class-gentry households in their use of antiseptic cleaning products. The local chemist's stock included a variety of antiseptic products that demonstrates their availability to all residents. It should be noted that both households that

---

33 Graham 2005.
34 Harris 2019.

35 Martyr 2002, 97.

Table 7.2 Identified categories of medicine bottles in the 2019 study on patent medicine bottles from Parramatta archaeological sites. Source: Harris 2019, 31.

Medicine category	Description
Gin/schnapps	While in the 21st century gin/schnapps is solely an alcoholic beverage, gin was originally a distilled herbal remedy containing juniper berry extract. It was used as a treatment for kidney disorders and subsequently included in many folk remedies, most notably mixed with quinine to combat the symptoms of malaria. During the late 19th century, schnapps was aggressively advertised in Australian newspapers for its medicinal properties.
Chemist	Flint glass dispensary types and those embossed with the names of local chemists – in the 18th and 19th centuries, flint glass was made from virtually pure quartz rock (calcined flint) to obtain the highest quality glass with no impurities that might contaminate the contents.
Pharmaceutical	These are bottles from reputable pharmaceutical laboratories that developed and manufactured both prescription and non-prescription medicine. These bottles were identified by embossed branding for the companies, which quite often occurs on the base of bottles.
Generic	Glassworks factories produced generic bottle shapes for use by chemists and proprietary medicine manufacturers. These shapes were identified from bottle manufacturers' catalogues.
Poisons	Topical medicine bottles identified by the embossment "Not to be Taken". This was to prevent accidental (or deliberate) oral consumption.
Patent and proprietary	These bottles were identified by branded trade-marked embossments.
Chinese	Small rectangular vials referred to by some as "opium bottles". They contained Chinese herbal remedies (only one site had a known Chinese component).

Table 7.3 Categories of medical complaints and relative frequencies identified in the 2019 patent medicine study area. Source: Harris 2019, 32.

Complaint	Relative frequency (%)	Complaint	Relative frequency (%)
Cure-all (excluding schnapps)	45.2	Ointment	0.7
Constipation	12.5	Supplement	0.7
Constipation/worms	10.5	Infection	0.3
Cough	9.8	Germs	0.3
Indigestion	5.7	Fainting	0.3
Pain	3.4	Denture cleaner	0.3
Antiseptic	3	Skin disease	0.3
Teething	2	Urinary infection	0.3
Coughs/colds	2	Back pain	0.3
Wounds/sores	1	Hair loss	0.3
Hair restorative	0.7		

7 The archaeology of personal health and social reforms

Table 7.4 Relative frequencies of medicine bottle types indentified in the 2019 patent medicine study in Parramatta. Source: Harris 2019, 31.

Case study site number	Address	Social class	Chemist (%)	Chinese (%)	Generic (%)	Patent (%)	Poison (%)	Prescription (%)	Schnapps (%)	Minimum Item Count
3	45 Macquarie St	Middle	10.6		18.4	25.6	0.5	8.2	36.7	207
7	2 George St	Working	14.5		20			9.1	56.4	55
1	4 George St	Middle	14.7	1.1	39.5	10	3.2	6.8	24.7	190
	97–99 Argyle St	Working	4		16	52		16	12	25
4	2 Taylor St	Middle	12.1	3.4	36.2	22.4	1.7	1.7	22.4	58
8	109 George St	Middle/gentry	17.6		5.9	29.4			47.1	34
6	100 George St	Middle/gentry	4.1		50.3	5.3	4.1		36.1	169
	Residential Total		10.7	0.5	32	15.9	2	5.4	33.5	738
	Parramatta Hospital	Surgeon's quarters	66.7			11.1			22.2	9
	41 George Street	Woolcott's dispensary	46.4		33.1	15.1	1.6		3.9	774

used antiseptics had a familial association with medical professionals, who would have been well informed on the newly developed "germ theory".

The inclusion of data on patent medicines sold at Woolcott's dispensary, the only recorded chemist's shop in Parramatta before the establishment of the 1876 New South Wales Register of Druggists and Chemists, added a layer of comparative analysis in that it demonstrated the availability of products in the over-the-counter market. Also, the presence of schnapps bottles in the shop's artefact assemblage suggests that some chemists sold the beverage as medicine. Not considered in the study is the observation that middle-class gentry, middle-class and working-class households used compounded medicines, most likely obtained from the local chemist. Whether these results speak to the frequency and severity of ailments and illness within individual households, or simply consumer choice, cannot be determined. Either the residents of the middle-class gentry households were healthier than those from middle-class and working-class households or they chose to self-medicate their ailments with patent medicines.

Mould, water pollution and patent medicines

Poor drainage in low-lying areas of Parramatta and an increasingly polluted water supply resulted in adverse medical conditions. Examination of artefacts from the archaeological collections of sites in the case study provides an opportunity to determine if these collections can contribute to understanding the effects of these harmful environmental conditions upon the residents of Parramatta. This undertaking can be achieved by analysing labelled patent medicine bottles, jars, vials and pots.

Implementing this analysis first required the identification of the ailments that are indicative of exposure to mould and polluted water supplies and the medicines used in the 19th century to treat their symptoms. Allergic reactions to mould have commonly manifested symptoms of skin or respiratory conditions or both, and can also include inflammatory symptoms that are characteristic of rheumatoid arthritis.[36] Typically, skin conditions range from rashes to dry skin and scaling, and symptoms of respiratory ailments include persistent coughs, congestion and a runny nose.[37] Contaminated water was potentially encountered through drinking, cooking, bathing, washing laundry and swimming. Ingesting tainted water causes gastrointestinal problems of varying degrees, depending upon the contaminating agents. Bathing and swimming in contaminated water can lead to infectious eye diseases, such as conjunctivitis or trachoma contracted from parasites and bacteria in the water; left untreated these lead to blindness.

General medicine categories to treat these symptoms include ointments, emulsions, cough syrups and elixirs, and purgatives. Ointments are a conventional treatment for topical allergic reactions to mould and contaminated water; they are applied to soothe and heal rashes. Emulsions are applied to relieve pain and inflammation of joints. Cough syrups and elixirs are taken to clear up respiratory distress. Purgatives are the most common remedies administered to treat ailments associated with ingestion of polluted water, including laxatives, salts, fluid magnesia and castor oil.

The availability of patent medicines in Parramatta is documented in the archaeological collection from Woolcott's dispensary.[38] This chemist's shop offered 30 branded products to treat numerous ailments including coughs, constipation, teething, muscle pain, respiratory problems, indigestion, hair loss and even liniments for veterinary ailments. While all the categories of medicines pertinent to this mould and pollution study were found in the case-study site assemblages, several limitations hindered the analysis of adverse effects of environmental contamination. The first limitation is the paucity of patent medicine bottles in the study (Table 7.4). Second, the principal manner to identify specific medicine containers is their labelling. Paper labels were common on all types of bottles throughout the 19th century; these labels generally do not survive in the archaeological record. Embossed labelling became increasingly more common from the second quarter of the 19th century and this type of labelling does endure. Consequently, all medicine bottles identified in this study are embossed-labelled bottles. All embossed-labelled bottles were recovered from features that post-date 1860 (sites 3–6, 8) and all but one have manufacturing date ranges that also post-date 1860 (Table 7.5). No labelled patent medicine bottles were recovered from assemblages for sites 1, 2, 7 and the Halfpenny occupation (1790–1830) at site 6. Products are identified by their embossed labels, and were researched for temporal information and to identify products marketed as treatments for the ailments described above (Table 7.6). Finally, these medications have multiple applications, and it cannot be definitively stated that they were administered for the sole purpose of alleviating symptoms associated with environmental contamination.

Personal hygiene and grooming

As previously demonstrated, cleanliness was a fundamental middle-class value. Personal hygiene, as a part of cleanliness, is a contributing factor to good health. Attitudes towards personal hygiene progressively changed during the 19th century. While research into some hygiene practices of individuals

---

36 Pirhonen, Nevalainen et al. 1996; M. Richards, Hyde and Williams 1956.
37 Prester 2011, 375.

38 Carney 1996.

Table 7.5 Patent medicines from case-study sites used for the treatment of symptoms of environmental contamination.

Medicine type	Ailment	Site 3	Site 4	Site 5	Site 6	Site 8
Cough	Respiratory distress	1				
Eye ointment	Conjunctivitis			1		
Digestive	Nausea/dyspepsia	1				
Purgative	Constipation	3	3		1	2
Emulsions	Muscle pain/arthritis	1		4		
Ointment	Rash	2	1			

Table 7.6 Patent medicine treatments from case-study sites that were used to combat symptoms of mould and water pollution.

Medicine type	Product name	First manufactured	Adjusted date range (date adjusted to include datable bottle attributes)	
Cough remedy	Powell's Balsam of Aniseed	1843	1843	
Laxative	Bishop's Granulated Citrate of Magnesia	1857	1857	1915
Laxative	California Fig Syrup Co	1878	1920	1970
Laxative	Dinneford's Fluid Magnesia	1846	1880	1930
Laxative	J.C. Eno's Salts	1876	1880	
Laxative	Morse's Indian Root Pills	1835	1920	
Laxative	Nujol	1901	1920	1940
Laxative	Hora & Co Castor Oil	1860	1860	1920
Muscle pain/ rheumatoid arthritis remedy	St Jakob's Oil	1878	1878	1900
Muscle pain/ rheumatoid arthritis remedy	Doan's Pills	1899	1899	1920
Muscle pain/ rheumatoid arthritis remedy	Elliman's Embrocation	1847	1847	1920
Ointment	Vaseline	1872	1920	
Ointment	Josephson's Australian Ointment	1866	1866	1900

cannot be ascertained from historical documentation, the archaeological record includes artefacts that further understanding of personal hygiene practices (ablutions, oral hygiene and grooming). Analysis data, shown in Tables 7.7 and 7.8, indicate that personal hygiene at the turn of the 19th century was limited to basic sanitation functions but, by the second quarter of the 19th century, increased oral hygiene practices were observed.

Ablutions

Bathing practices until the mid-19th century were limited to a periodic sponge bath and were primarily a matter of appearance. Daily sponge bathing was uncommon in middle-class and working-class homes until after the mid-1800s. *Cassell's Household Guide* of the 1870s advised sponging oneself daily. As Table 7.7 shows, the use of ewers and washbasins in the case-study assemblages increased during the 19th century. Full-body bathing was a minority pursuit in the 19th century, even among society's wealthiest – once a week was ample.[39] Governor King's bathhouse, built in 1822, was a rare example of full-body bathing practices in Parramatta. In New South Wales, changing attitudes towards bathing were largely due to aggressive health reform campaigns in the 1850s, campaigns that included the 1886 *Parramatta Public Baths Act*, culminating with the construction and maintenance of the riverside Centennial Baths.[40]

---

39   Jackson 2014, 136.
40   Levine 1996, 1186.

Cleanliness is next to godliness

Table 7.7 Quantitative data tabulated for personal hygiene-related artefacts ordered by feature dates.

Site number	Address	Feature type	Feature number	Chamber-pot (%)	Ewer (%)	Washbasin (%)	Soap dish (%)	Toothbrush (%)	Toothpaste (%)	Begin date (*Terminus post quem*)	End date (*Terminus anti quem*)
7	2 George St	Cellar	3957	9						1800	1850
2	15 Macquarie St	Dam	10350	3		2				1800	1835
1	4 George St	Cesspit	6024	7			1	4		1820	1860
1	4 George St	Cesspit	6039		1					1830	1870
8	109 George St	Pit	5073	6	3	4		1	1	1820	1860
3	45 Macquarie St	Well	775	3	1				3	1860	1890
6	100 George St	Well	2417	8	1	2			1	1860	1900
6	100 George St	Cesspit	2206					3		1865	1930
6	100 George St	Cesspit	2369	3		1		6		1870	1930
6	100 George St	Cesspit	2370	1	1	1				1875	1920
4	2 Taylor St	Cistern	4702	4		1	1			1890	1920
5	13–15 Taylor St	Cistern	147	3		2			1	1900	1935

7 The archaeology of personal health and social reforms

Table 7.8 Relative frequencies calculated for personal hygiene artefacts for case-study sites.

Site No	Address	Feature type	Feature number	Chamber-pot (%)	Ewer (%)	Washbasin (%)	Soap dish (%)	Toothbrush (%)	Toothpaste (%)	Total features
7	2 George St	Cellar	3957	1.97						457
2	15 Macquarie St	Dam	10350	0.12		0.08				2511
1	4 George St	Cesspit	6024	0.27			0.04	0.15		2631
1	4 George St	Cesspit	6039		5.26					19
8	109 George St	Pit	5073	2.42	1.21	1.61		0.4	0.4	248
3	45 Macquarie St	Well	775	0.12	0.03				0.12	2995
6	100 George St	Well	2417	0.27	0.03	0.07			0.03	2935
6	100 George St	Cesspit	2206					0.28		1089
6	100 George St	Cesspit	2369	0.26		0.09		0.53		1137
6	100 George St	Cesspit	2370	0.08	0.08	0.08				1247
4	2 Taylor St	Cistern	4702	1.3		0.33	0.33			307
5	13–15 Taylor St	Cistern	147	0.84		0.56			0.28	358

71

The use of chamber-pots was ubiquitous throughout the 19th century in Parramatta, as the municipal sewerage scheme was not completed until 1910. Residents relied upon these vessels to accumulate night soil and later be disposed of in available cesspits.

Oral hygiene

Oral hygiene has been practised for centuries, including proactive teeth and tongue cleaning, and reactive measures such as filling, lamenting and extraction. Until the 19th century, one of the most common proactive oral hygiene practices to clean one's teeth was with aromatic twigs and salt or chalk. Rarely do these items survive in the archaeological record, so our knowledge of their use is limited. Toothbrushes were first used in Britain during the 17th century, but, until they were commercially produced in the 19th century, they were primarily used by the upper classes.[41] Attitudes towards oral hygiene practices also started to improve by the mid-1800s, fostered in part by the availability of toothbrushes and tooth powders or toothpaste, and in part by changing dietary habits that resulted in increased tooth decay due to higher consumption rates of refined sugar.[42]

During the first few years of New South Wales settlement, the only recorded use of sugar was by Royal Naval surgeons, presumably for compounding medicines.[43] Contracted shipments of sugar arrived with each successive convict ship, but sugar availability most likely improved when by 1791 it was found that crops of sugarcane thrived on Norfolk Island.[44] By 1796 many convicts had served their sentences and, as paid labourers, were desirous of better clothing and a few more "little luxuries". This prompted the governor to request increases in the shipment of tea and sugar.[45] Moderately successful attempts were made to grow sugarcane near Port Macquarie in 1821 and the first sugarcane refinery, built in Sydney in 1842, processed imported sugar.[46] The Australian sugar industry developed significantly between 1864 and 1884 in a vast area stretching from Grafton in New South Wales to Mossman in Queensland.[47] By the last quarter of the 19th century, there was a ready supply of sugar to the colony.

Throughout the 18th century and much of the 19th century, teeth were extracted by barbers or dentists. The first dentist arrived in New South Wales by 1814. Before this, the only orthodox dental treatment available in the colony was essential emergency services carried out by a Colonial Medical Service member. In 1829, surgeon and dentist Dr Henry Jeanneret, a recent immigrant, published his treatise *Hints for the preservation of teeth*, which was the first book in the colony on preventative dentistry. By the mid-1800s dentistry was officially recognised in Britain with the first British *Dental Act* enacted in 1878.[48] The first *Dentistry Act* in New South Wales, enacted in 1900, required the registration of qualified dental practitioners. Qualifications ranged from university diplomas to two-year apprenticeships or passing the New South Wales Dentistry Board's examination. Six Parramatta dentists had registered by 1902.[49]

In their archaeological study, *Diet and dental caries in post-medieval London*, Mant and Roberts present an in-depth analysis of the link between diet and the increase of dental caries (cavities) during the 18th and 19th centuries. They cite numerous works when they make the statement: "Many researchers posit that an increased dependence upon carbohydrates and the introduction of refined sugars have increased the rates of caries diachronically for many human groups".[50]

In 18th-century Britain, the annual consumption of refined sugar increased by 100 per cent during the first half of the century (from 1.8 to 3.6 kilograms) and by 400 per cent by the end of the century (8.2 kilograms). This rise is linked with the increase in tea drinking, and with the consumption of associated sweet bakery treats. During the 19th century, sugar consumption doubled again. Two factors contributed to this increase: availability and affordability as a result of the lowering, and eventual removal, of tariffs on the commodity.[51] The study goes on to indicate that improved refinement techniques in flour also contributed to the increase in dental caries. They resulted in an upsurge in the popularity of white bread, which is more cariogenic than the darker rye and barley varieties.

Toothbrushes were recovered from three household assemblages, four recovered from the middle-class McRoberts household (site 1), one from the middle-class gentry Hassall household (site 8) and nine from the middle-class gentry Byrnes household (site 6), with toothpaste pots recovered from only the Hassall and Byrnes household (Figure 7.1). While no toothbrushes were recovered from the middle-class assemblages on Taylor Street, there was one zinc toothpaste tube recovered from an early 20th-century deposit at 15 Taylor Street (site 5).

Due to the absence of dental remains in collections for this case study and the lack of dental and dentition studies in Australia, we must rely upon British studies for comparative temporal and social-class data from 19th-century sites. According to Mant and Roberts, several diachronic studies found an increase in rates of dental caries over time, and there were no significant differences in the rates of caries by social status.[52] Mant and Robert's

---

41 M. Freeman 2001.
42 Mattick 2010, 8.
43 *Historical Records of New South Wales* Series 1, vol. 1 1914, 58, 88.
44 *Historical Records of New South Wales* Series 1, vol. 1 1914, 234.
45 *Historical Records of New South Wales* Series 1, vol. 1 1914, 594.
46 Australian Cane Farmers Association 2006.
47 Griggs 2011, 1.

48 Fricker, Kiley et al. 2011, 93.
49 Office of Minister of Public Health 1903.
50 Mant and Roberts 2014, 201.
51 Mant and Roberts 2014, 201.
52 Mant and Roberts 2014, 196.

7 The archaeology of personal health and social reforms

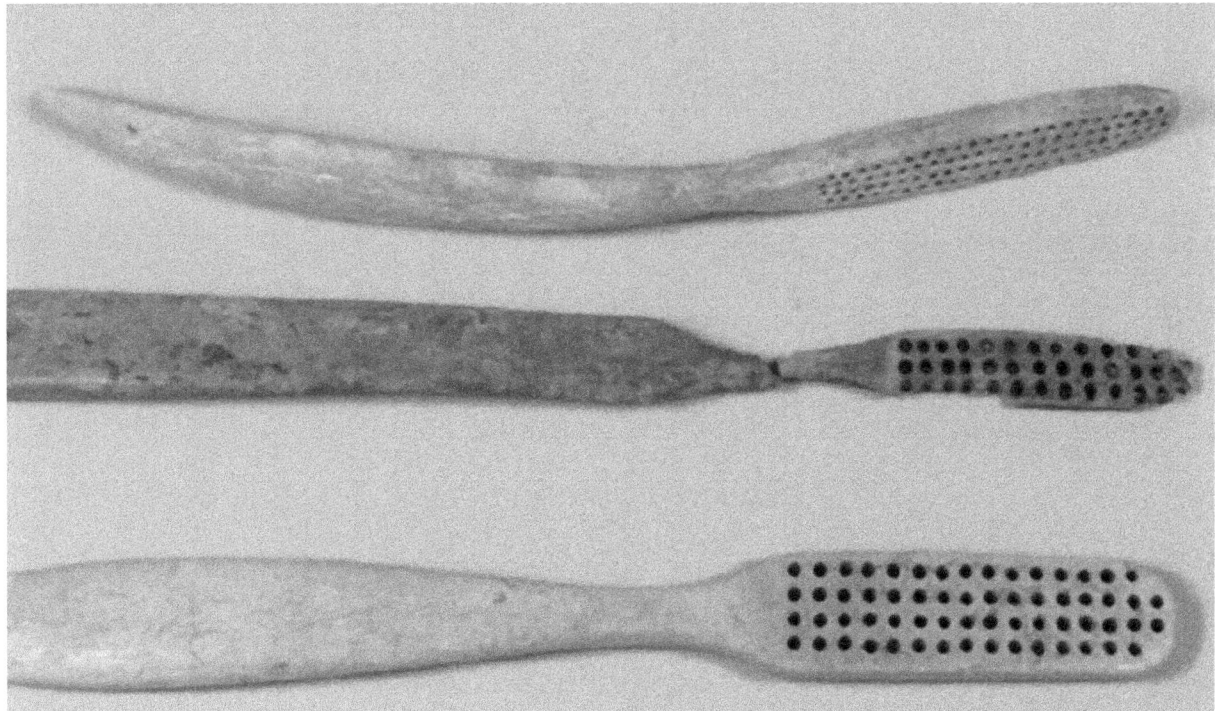

Figure 7.1 Toothbrushes recovered from 4 George Street (site 1). Source: Stocks 2009, 39.

study found a high prevalence of tooth loss among both classes, suggesting a non-class-specific preference for removing teeth rather than choosing the more expensive option of fillings.[53] Unfortunately, their study does not include a comparison of dental fillings between social classes. Identification differences in social-class approaches to dentistry in New South Wales present an opportunity for future research by examining personal accounts recorded in diaries, letters and memoirs.

Laundry and household cleanliness

One aspect of personal hygiene not readily addressed in the archaeological record is evidence for washing of clothing. As previously discussed, fresh water was initially plentiful in early Parramatta but quickly became an issue for settlers, as supply would have come from wells, been collected in cisterns from run-off or been hauled in from the river or municipal standpipes. Not every working-class family lived in abject poverty, but most struggled to wash themselves and their clothes. Middle-class families fared much better as they employed servants who did household laundry, cooking and cleaning, had sufficient fuel to heat the water as well as plenty of soap and whitening. Some even hired an additional washerwoman to assist on washday. They would have had copper boilers with a laundry dolly. A laundry dolly is a wooden rod with a crossway handle at the top and six legs radiating out of the base. Using the dolly involved a combination of a downward and rotational movement to move the laundry around in a swirling and twisting motion. As the century progressed, a mangle (hand-turned washing machine) was used. Furthermore, washing activities were typically conducted in a designated outbuilding. While evidence of appropriate outbuildings was identified for all case-study sites, no evidence was found that explicitly links these structures to laundry activities.

Even convicts were vigilant about their ablutions and laundry. The March 1826 Grand Jury review of the Parramatta Female Factory states that the women were poorly clothed and shod. However, it also stated that habits of cleanliness were evidenced by the laundry facilities, in which the linen of 160 women was washed weekly.[54]

An extension of personal hygiene was household cleanliness, as it affects personal health. The awareness of the newly accepted "germ theory" is evidenced here by cleaning products found in the late 19th-century to early 20th-century assemblages. The middle-class gentry Byrnes household assemblage and middle-class tenant household assemblage at 15 Taylor Street included bottles for cleaning products, such as disinfectants, ammonia, Lysol and carbolic acid, that demonstrate the family's awareness of germs and the importance of a clean home environment.

Personal grooming

Personal grooming is a subset of personal hygiene that relates to the physical presence of a clean and ordered body. In the Victorian era, body modification practices,

---

53 Mant and Roberts 2014, 197.

54 *Sydney Gazette and New South Wales Advertiser* 3 March 1825, 3.

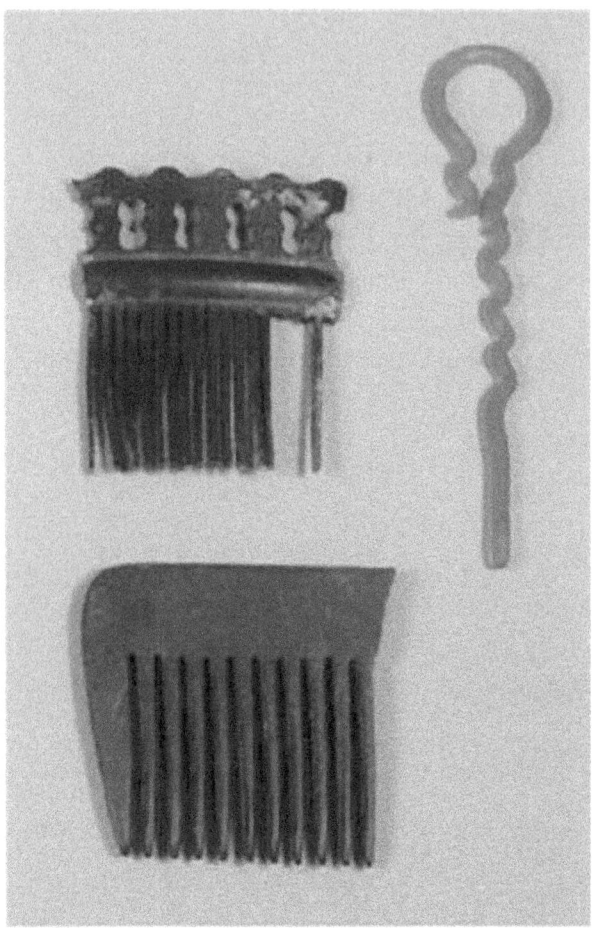

Figure 7.2 Hair combs recovered from 4 George Street (site 1). Source: Stocks 2009, 39.

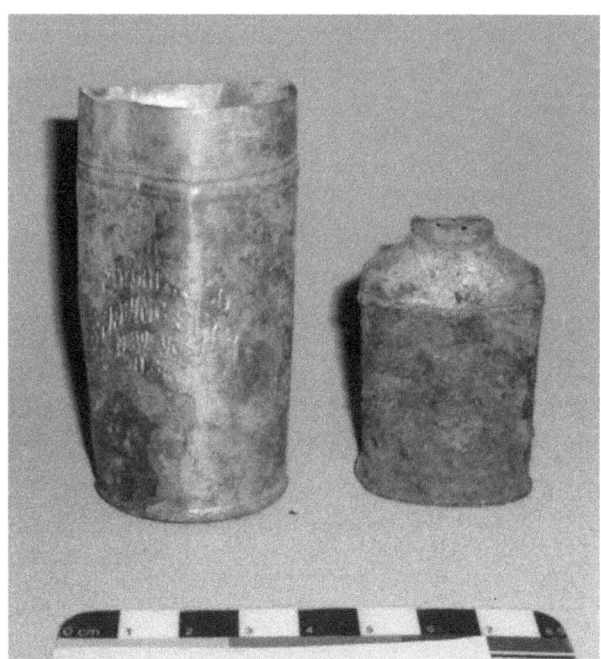

Figure 7.3 Shaving product tins recovered from 13–15 Taylor Street (site 5). Source: GML Heritage 2015: 92.

such as shaving, hairstyling (dying, cutting and combing) and manicuring nails, represent visual ways of portraying the illusion of cleanliness. The use of fragrances fosters this illusion by masking body odours. In the archaeological record, grooming items typically consist of grooming tools and bottles that contained associated products. Tools include those for grooming hair (combs, brushes and scissors) and shaving (razor, shaving mugs and brushes) (Figures 7.2 and 7.3). Some combs were of the plain sort used for grooming while others were ornamental combs that were used for styling. Shaving mugs were used mainly in conjunction with a straight razor, shaving brush and a hardened shaving soap disc. Mugs, brushes and soap were used in combination with a straight razor before the patent of the safety razor in 1887. Commercial containers include products for hair treatment (tonics, restoratives, pomades and dyes), skin products (creams and lotions), manicuring tools and products (cuticle treatments and polish) and fragrances (perfume, cologne, powders and lavender water).

Enhancement cosmetics (make-up) were not readily available, as respectable ladies wore no make-up and only ladies of questionable occupations used them.

Information on the availability of grooming tools and products is mostly limited to notices of sale in newspaper advertisements. One of the earliest was an 1821 import notice by Mr Josephson of Pitt Street, Sydney, which includes a long list of items including:

> Windsor, palm, violet, rose, and shaving soaps; wash balls; rouge, in pots; pomatum; rose and jessamine oils; lavender, honey, pearl, and rose waters; milk of roses; cream of roses; curling fluid; tooth powder; vegetable dye; pocket, tail, and crop combs; ivory tooth combs; patent hair, cloth, tooth, and shaving brushes; razor strops; pewter and wooden shaving boxes, &c ...[55]

As Table 7.9 shows, personal grooming artefacts recovered from the sites consist of fragrances used to give the body a pleasant smell and items used for hair grooming and shaving that helped to portray cleanliness. Fragrances were recovered from most sites and no discernible difference between social classes was observed but lavender water was only found in the assemblages for the two earliest sites (2 George Street and 15 Macquarie Street).

Shaving-related artefacts were recovered from the two middle-class tenanted households on Taylor Street. During the mid-19th century, beards became fashionable and were a sign of masculinity, and the absence of a beard was a sign of physical and moral weakness.[56] Around the turn of the 20th-century changes in Australian facial-hair fashion resulted in a decline in the popularity of beards, and facial hair was generally limited to moustaches and

---

55 *Sydney Gazette and New South Wales Advertiser* 11 August 1821, 2.
56 Peterkin 2001.

7 The archaeology of personal health and social reforms

Table 7.9 Relative frequencies calculated for personal grooming artefacts for case-study sites.

Site number	Address	Feature type	Feature number	Comb (%)	Hairpin (%)	Lavender water (%)	Perfume (%)	Shaving cream (%)	Shaving mug (%)	Talcum powder (%)	Total	Total feature
2	15 Macquarie St	Dam	10350			0.04					1	2511
3	45 Macquarie St	Well	775	0.1			0.1				8	2995
7	2 George St	Cellar	3927			0.3	0.6				3	457
1	4 George St	Cesspit	6024	0.08			0.08				4	2631
8	109 George St	Pit	5073	0.4							1	248
6	100 George St	Cesspit	2206		0.09		0.09				2	1089
6	100 George St	Cesspit	2369				0.09				1	1137
6	100 George St	Cesspit	2370				0.08				1	1247
4	2 Taylor St	Cistern	4702				1.3		0.33		5	307
5	13–15 Taylor St	Cistern	147				1.4	0.28		0.28	7	358

goatees. Dating from the late 19th century to early 20th century, shaving accessories, present in the two Taylor Street assemblages, are consistent with shaving practices of the day.

Vices – patterns of alcohol and tobacco consumption

Drinking and smoking habits are behavioural conventions influenced by public attitudes. Alcohol and tobacco have been an integral part of Australian culture since the First Fleet arrived in 1788.[57] In a colony with little currency until 1800, spirits (rum, brandy and gin) were one commodity commonly used to pay convict workers and pipe smoking was one of the few leisure privileges afforded to convicts.[58] As New South Wales evolved from a convict settlement to a frontier colony, so did its attitudes towards alcohol consumption and tobacco smoking. Simply put, the view of middle-class men, such as Magistrate Rev. Marsden, on smoking was that it led to excessive drinking, which in turn led to criminal activities.

Political and social reforms for alcohol and tobacco differ in their history and evolution. Information on these reforms comes from the historical record. The reforms are individually discussed below. The historical record gives insight into the political actions taken to contend with these issues, the statistics that reflect these actions and the social activism responsible for initiating these actions. What we see is the public face of temperance reform. One means of understanding the private face of temperance is to look at the archaeological record for evidence of the individual's response to these reforms by examining the rubbish they left behind and interpreting the data to assess if individuals practised social reforms within the walls of their homes.

Alcohol

As Horton's widely accepted "anxiety theory" suggests, the "primary purpose of alcohol in any society was to reduce anxiety in an unstable social environment".[59] Early colonial New South Wales was most assuredly an unstable social environment. Contributing physical environmental influences, such as a dry, hot climate and a different ecological setting, added to this perturbation. Convicts and officials alike drank to escape the reality of the harsh life that confronted them.[60] While perhaps exaggerated, Colonel David Collins observed in 1793:

> The passion for liquor was so predominant among the people that it operated like a mania, there being nothing that they would not risk to obtain it; and while spirits were to be had, those who did any extra labour refused to be paid in money or in any other article than spirits.[61]

Archaeological evidence for alcohol consumption

The archaeological record is rich in data with the potential to contribute statistics on alcohol consumption patterns, yet archaeologists generally fail to address the impact of alcohol on society. Historical documents and analyses contribute a wealth of knowledge on public alcohol consumption patterns. However, archaeology has the potential to provide data for a comparative study on in-home drinking practices.

In the archaeological record, evidence of in-home alcohol consumption consists mostly of glass and ceramic bottles. Analysis of these bottles produces patterns of consumption that further our knowledge of individual responses to social reforms. Identification of commercial alcohol containers is key to the analytical process. Bottles have distinct shapes that make for quick identification of the content. As Lindsey states, "liquor bottle diversity is staggeringly complex in depth and variety".[62] A type series to streamline the classification of Parramatta alcohol bottles is organised into five basic categories: beer/wine; champagne; spirits; ginger beer; and schnapps (Table 7.10). In addition, there are situations where a bottle displays many characteristics of an alcohol bottle, but insufficient identification markers are available to pinpoint its specific category placement, and it is categorised as an unspecified alcohol container. As aerated water bottles are included as an alternative beverage, they, too, were added to the type series.

One of the common issues in establishing a type series for bottles is defining the parameters used in classification. Here, a basic form/function type series is used; it is not designed to categorise manufacturing attributes that establish a bottle's temporal placement, which was established during the previous artefact analysis conducted for consultancy reports.

The archaeology of alcohol consumption allows investigation beyond the historical documentation to answer alternative questions and develop alternate interpretations that "do not rely on historical documents or documentary historians as final arbiters of meaningful or accurate history".[63] Historian Matt Allen's chronicles of alcohol regulation supply a background for controls on alcohol sales in New South Wales. Dingle's statistics on alcohol consumption in New South Wales allow a comparative study with the archaeological record for Parramatta (Figure 7.4).[64] Parramatta's archaeological record, based on statistics drawn from sites in the case

---

57 Blocker, Fahey and Tyrrell 2003, 75; Walker 1980, 11.
58 Walker 1984, 9.
59 Blocker, Fahey and Tyrrell 2003, 45; Gusfield 1986; Horton 1943, 223; Smith 2008.
60 Dingle 1980, 237.

61 In W.S. Campbell 1932, 86.
62 Lindsey 2010.
63 Little 1994, 8.
64 Dingle 1980.

7 The archaeology of personal health and social reforms

Table 7.10 Illustrations, photographs and descriptions of alcohol bottle types identified in the case study.

Alcohol bottle type	Illustration	Description
Late 18th to early 19th-century British types		British cylindrical beer/wine bottle shapes evolved over time. Late 18th-century shapes were dip-moulded and characterised by a rounded heel (some with basal sag). Applied glass for finish consisting of a separate lip and string-rim applications. There was no standardised volume.
British imperial wine and wine types		British cylindrical imperial beer/wine and wine shapes resulted from the standardisation of volume in the 1824 *British Imperial Weights and Measures Act*, which served to standardise bottle sizes, but the general shape remained the same. These types are dip-moulded and 3-piece-moulded with abrupt heels and applied glass for finish consisted of separate lip and string-rim applications and a single application for a form-tooled finish.
Champagne/ burgundy type		Champagne style bottles have a tapering neck/body, rounded heel with a deep push up and large boss on base, sloped shoulder and applied glass for a string-rim finish.
Union Oval Flask Type		A spirit bottle, oval shaped flask termed a Union oval flask by bottle manufacturers and a pint flask by others is characterised by a flattened elliptical shape with a body that tapers slightly from shoulder to heel.[a]
Schnapps – Late 18th to 20th century		The dip-moulded blown Dutch gin bottle is a common style found in Australian archaeological collections. In addition to the square flat-sided body profile, the body tapers from shoulder to heel. The characteristic 4-point resting place heel, evidenced on many bottles from Australian archaeological contexts, was introduced in the 17th century, well before the first Europeans settled in the colony.[b] This bottle style was manufactured in European countries, such as Germany and the Netherlands, throughout the 19th century.
Schnapps – Mid-19th century		The development of the 2- and 3-piece mould in the second quarter of the 19th century altered the shape of most schnapps bottles. The body was no longer tapered and the heel was flat. The lip was applied and form tooled.
Ginger beer		Stoneware ginger beer bottles had a cylindrical shape and thick finish; in early manufacture, the shoulder was rounded, and the vessel was lead-glazed. By the mid-19th century, these bottles exhibited a sharp shoulder and were commonly salt-glazed. The same body shape continued through to the 20th century with a slightly concave dip above the shoulder, a variety of glaze types and they often exhibited transfer-printed product labelling.
Dates for stoneware ginger beer bottles	c.1820s 1850s–1860s 1900s *terminus post quem*	

a Lindsey 2010.
b McNulty 2004, 24.

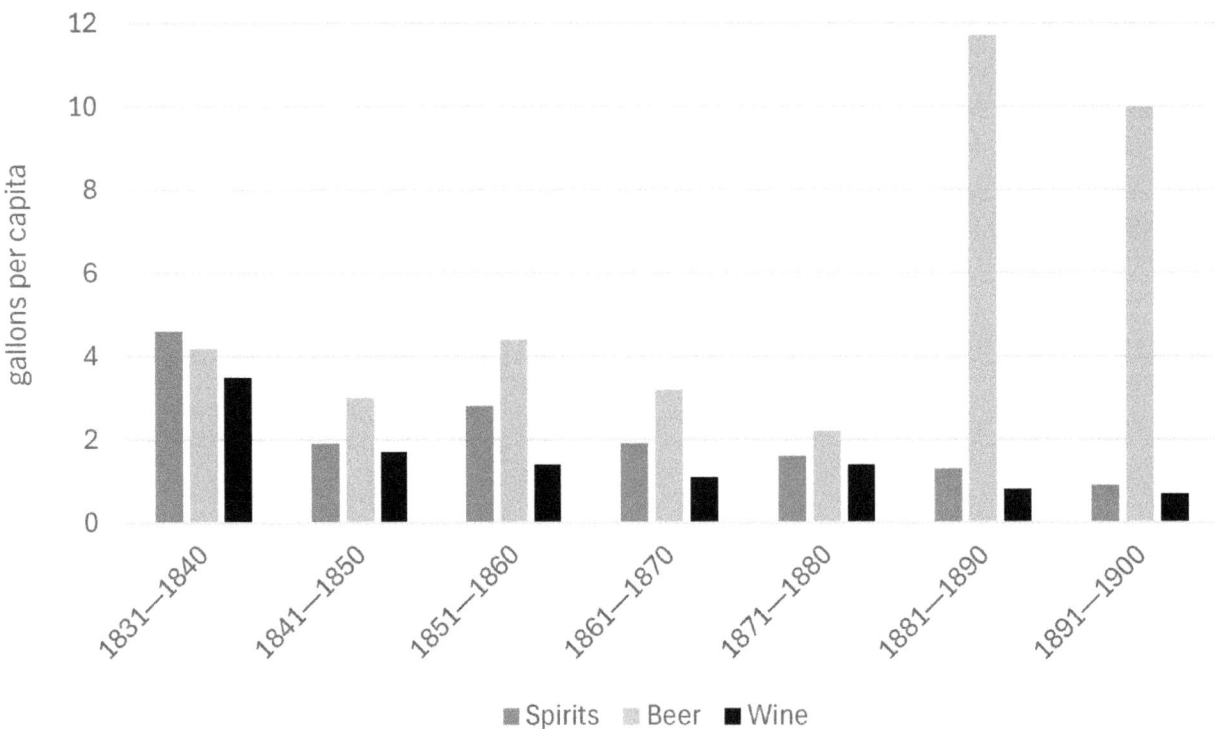

Figure 7.4 Graphic representation of Dingle's per capita annual alcohol consumption for New South Wales.

study, has the potential to reveal more than just relative frequency of alcohol consumption: there is the potential to demonstrate consistencies and changes in the types of alcohol consumed, and potentially even a shift in preference to non-alcoholic beverages.

Dingle's per capita consumption statistics have been calculated from data contained in the annual Statistical Registers of each colony, and he presents these as averages of alcohol consumed by gallons and by decades (1831–1900). These statistics are divided into three categories: spirits, beer and wine. In Parramatta's archaeological record, the statistics are presented as relative frequencies of alcohol categories based on identified bottle forms: beer; beer or wine; champagne type; gin or schnapps; and spirit bottles. To make the two sets of data comparable, some conversions are required. Firstly, Dingle's categories are converted to relative frequency for each type as they related to total alcohol consumption, and beer and wine categories are combined. Secondly, for the case-study statistics for beer and wine, champagne and beer categories are combined (as beer and wine) and spirits, gin and schnapps categories are combined (as spirits).

A limitation of Dingle's data is that before 1881, it did not include locally-brewed beer. Beer was a traditional drink of rural life and Parramatta was still very much a rural settlement during the first decades of the 19th century.[65] Prior to the 1855 arrival of the railway in Parramatta, transport networks were limited to overland wagons, making it challenging to transport beer any great distance from its point of manufacture. Therefore, there were local breweries in the Parramatta district that supplied beer to the local market, and Parramatta is located on a river with access to supply the downriver markets in Sydney. The earliest regional brewery was James Squire's (1793), which was established at Kissing Point, a riverfront location one mile east of Parramatta. By Squire's own account, the product of his first brewing efforts was small, made from hops he acquired from the supply ship *Daedalus*, but it is speculated that with the 1,200 lb of hops he obtained he could have produced 19,000 gallons of beer or roughly 4 gallons for each person living in the colony at that time.[66] During its first year of operation, the government-owned Parramatta Brewery (1804–1810) could produce 6,000 gallons of beer per month. Parramatta's population in 1804 was 1,900, which suggests the Parramatta Brewery on a monthly average was supplying 3.1 gallons of beer per capita.

For comparative purposes, the statistics for features in the Parramatta case study are organised chronologically (Table 7.11). Initial analysis of relative frequencies in both studies indicate that throughout the 70-year time span (used in Dingle's statistics) more beer and wine were consumed than spirits. Closer examination of statistics shows that in the Parramatta study relative frequencies for beer and wine are consistently higher

---

65 Lewis 1992, 6.

66 Allen 2013, 79; Deutsher 1999, 67.

7 The archaeology of personal health and social reforms

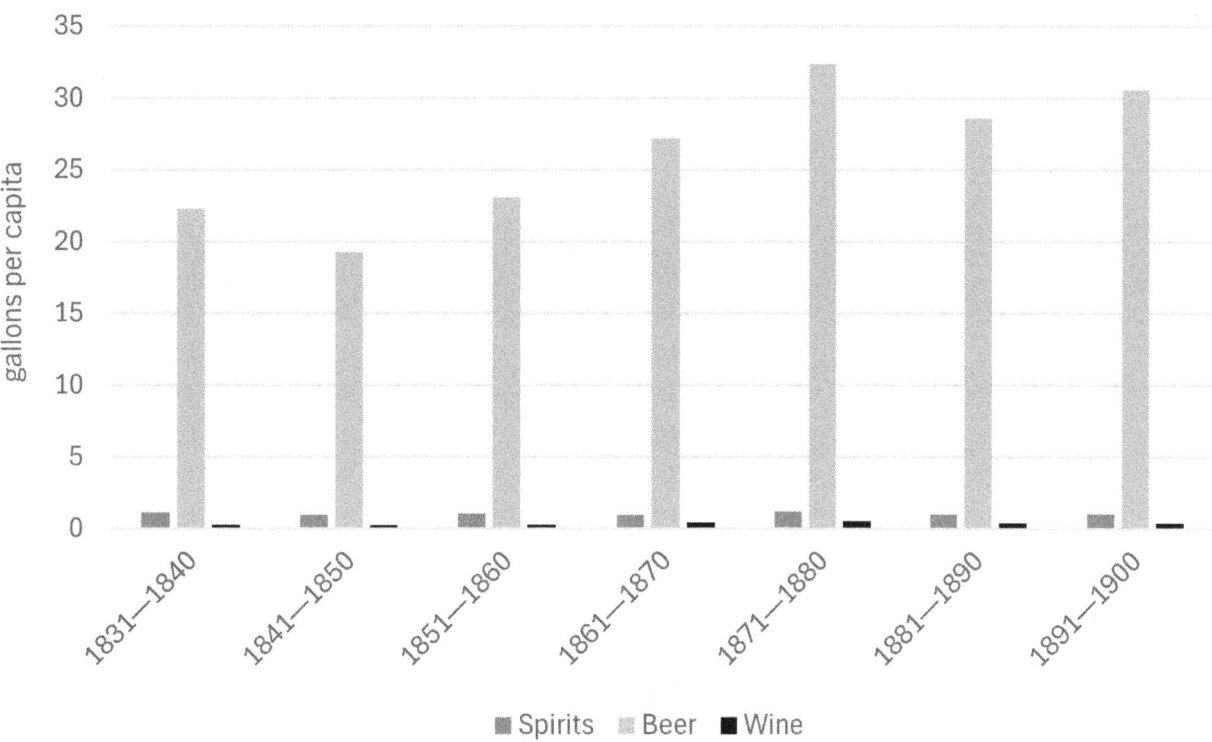

Figure 7.5 Graphic representation of Dingle's per capita alcohol consumption for Great Britain.

than Dingle's study, even with the 1881 inclusion of local beer consumption in his statistics.

As previously noted, New South Wales had its peak annual per capita consumption of spirits in the 1830s, which was more than four times higher than in Britain (Figures 7.4 and 7.5).[67] Like New South Wales, the annual per capita consumption of beer (by volume) in Great Britain was always higher than spirits throughout the 19th century.[68] Also, annual British beer consumption was consistently and substantially higher than in the colony. The peak period of per capita alcohol consumption was 1874–1876 (both spirits and beer).[69] The colony's per capita consumption of wine was always higher than in the UK, especially in the 1830s when 13 times more wine was consumed.

Analysis of aerated water and schnapps bottles contributes statistics on changes in alcohol consumption patterns not identified in the data discussed above. Both aerated waters and schnapps had their origins in medicine, both play a role in patterns of alcohol consumption and the temperance movement influenced both. Yet, each had a separate evolution, and each had a different role to play in colonial drinking patterns.

Schnapps

The increased influence of the temperance movement and the increased popularity of schnapps in the colony contributed to changing alcohol consumption attitudes. From the late 1830s, schnapps was marketed worldwide as a patent medicine. It presented people with the opportunity to consume alcoholic beverages in their homes while avoiding the disdain of neighbours, church members and temperance reformers.[70] Medicinal schnapps was officially introduced to the colonial markets in the 1860s, when Udolpho Wolfe launched an aggressive marketing campaign through many colonial newspapers. Avoiding the stigma associated with gin, Wolfe used the German word "schnapps" for his product.

A comparative analysis of alcoholic beverages shows a low relative frequency of schnapps bottles in feature assemblages that date before the 1860s and a noticeable increase in relative frequencies for schnapps bottles in most features that post-date 1860 (Table 7.11).

---

67 Blocker, Fahey and Tyrrell 2003, 75.
68 Wilson 1940, 332–3.
69 Webb 1913, 207.

70 Blocker, Fahey and Tyrrell 2003, 54.

Cleanliness is next to godliness

Table 7.11 Relative frequencies calculated for beverage types from features in case-study sites.

Site number	Address	Date range	Feature type	Alcohol (%)	Beer (%)	Beer and wine (%)	Champagne (%)	Gin and schnapps (%)	Spirits (%)	Total alcohol (%)	Aerated water (%)	Total Minimum Item Count
7	2 George St	1810–40s	Cellar			96.2	1.3	2.5		100		79
6	100 George St	1790–1830	Rubbish pit			100.0				100		2
2	15 Macquarie St	1823–41	Dam	20.0		73.3	6.7			100.0		15
1	4 George St	1820–60	Cesspit 6024			88.1	9.5	2.4		100.0		42
1	4 George St	1830–70	Cesspit 6039			66.7	33.3			100.0		3
8	109 George St	1860–80	Rubbish pit			84.6		2.6	7.7	94.9	5.1	39
3	45 Macquarie St	1860–90	Well	4.3		34.8	30.4	26.1	4.3	100.0		23
6	100 George St	1865–90	Cesspit 2370			66.7	8.3	16.7		91.7	8.3	12
6	100 George St	1865–1940	Cesspit 2206			25.0	25.0	25.0		75.0	25.0	4
6	100 George St	1865–1930	Cesspit 2369			77.8	11.1			88.9	11.1	9
4	2 Taylor St	1890–1920	Cistern			59.1	22.7		4.5	86.4	13.6	22
5	13–15 Taylor St	1900–30	Cistern	4.8	4.8	14.3	9.5	9.5	4.8	47.6	52.4	21

Non-alcoholic beverages: aerated water

While alcohol has been an important part of Australian culture since first settlement, all settlers, from ardent consumers of alcohol to teetotallers, had the need for lighter beverages, such as ginger beer and spruce to quench the thirst caused by Australia's hotter climate. Artificial manufacture of effervescing water was developed in the late 18th century and some accounts claimed it was a cure for scurvy.[71] When Dr Joseph Priestley discovered a means of artificially carbonating water, he published his process in a pamphlet in 1772.[72] This innovation led to aerated water's commercial packaging, but a commercial container for aerated water still proved a challenge. The pressure generated by the effervescing beverage necessitated packaging in bottles that could withstand the pressure. It was first packaged in existing stoneware bottle forms that were originally used for stout and beer; however, if the cork closures were not kept moist, the stoppers dried out, then shrank and the gas leaked out.[73] Round-bottom and pointed-bottom glass bottles were adopted to ensure that corks stayed moist, because they required the vessel to rest on its side when not open, which kept the cork moist. Unfortunately, the pressure of the gas within the bottle could still force the stopper out. The foremost factor for the increase of commercial production and bottling of aerated waters lay in improving bottle closures for glass bottles, which enabled the bottle to withstand the pressure while resting in a vertical position. Starting in the early 1860s there were many patents registered in Europe, Great Britain and the United States for aerated water bottle closures, opening the way for successful commercial manufacture.[74] The most successful patents were for bottles with internal stoppers such as Codd and Lamont patented forms.

The development of artificial carbonation and the subsequent improvements for bottle closures made aerated waters more readily available to the Australian market. As Parramatta grew, so did its aerated water industry. Between 1834 and 1925 there were 22 aerated water bottlers in Parramatta.[75] The first bottler was Edward Smith and during the next decade two more short-lived aerated water businesses were established. Between 1850 and 1860 two new businesses were established, three new businesses in the 1870s, four in the 1880s, five in the 1890s and five in the first quarter of the 20th century.[76] Bottles from these bottlers and those from nearby Sydney firms are frequently recovered during archaeological investigations of Parramatta sites.

Increased availability resulted in increased consumption. This increase is demonstrated through a simple dichotomous comparison of relative frequencies of alcohol bottles and aerated water bottles from case-study sites, as well as from features associated with two Parramatta public houses (inns) outside the case study (Table 7.12).[77] The two inns used in this comparison were located on Lot 19 on Church Street, Parramatta. The earliest was the Baker's Arms Inn (1830–1859), which moved to Parramatta's northern limits on Church Street at Albert Street in 1859. In 1860, the Lot 19 building became the Star Inn (1850s–1902).[78] The footprint of the building was demolished during the construction of a large 20th-century basement for the new Starr Hotel. Archaeological excavations located a sealed brick-lined cesspit associated with the Star Inn occupation at the rear boundary of the property and a circular rubbish pit along the northern boundary that was associated with the earlier Baker's Arms Inn occupation. These archaeological features remained in situ until the 2017 redevelopment of the site.[79]

Bottle forms (aerated water and alcohol) were identified and temporal placement was achieved through the documentation for bottle manufacturers, bottle patents and product bottlers, established using standard Australian references.[80] This comparison was limited to glass bottles because the stoneware bottle forms initially used for aerated waters were used simultaneously for stout and beer, making their specific use indeterminate. Date ranges for features were established during temporal analysis for all recovered artefact types. Furthermore, due to the varying assemblage sizes in each feature, each beverage type's deposit data are represented as relative frequencies.

From the 1830s, aerated waters gained increased popularity as refreshing beverages.[81] Yet Dingle's study indicates that a decline in the consumption of alcoholic beverages did not occur until the 1890s (Figure 7.4). A comparative analysis was undertaken to identify patterns of public and private alcohol and aerated water consumption to assess this change in preference for aerated water beverages in Parramatta. As Table 7.12 shows, no aerated water bottles were found in either the residential or public assemblages for much of the first half of the 19th century. During the second half of the 19th century, aerated water bottles were found in the assemblages and generally in increasing relative frequencies. While the development of artificially carbonated water, and development of required bottles and closures, made possible the rapid growth of the aerated water industry, obtainability is not the only factor that influenced the consumption patterns for aerated waters. Technological advancements alone do not explain the change in consumer choice. The decrease in the clean

---

71 Emmins 1991, 8–10.
72 Priestley 1772.
73 Munsey 2010.
74 Paul and Parmalee 1973, 3–10.
75 Harris 2021, 201; D. Jones 2009.
76 D. Jones 2009.
77 Harris 2019.
78 *Sydney Morning Herald* 8 December 1859, 3.
79 Miskella 2017, 50, 98.
80 Deutsher 1999; D. Jones 2009; Lindsey 2010; Munsey 1970.
81 Emmins 1991, 8–10.

Cleanliness is next to godliness

Table 7.12 Relative frequencies of alcohol and aerated water bottles recovered from case-study sites in chronological order.

Site number	Terminus post quem	Terminus anti quem	Address	Site type	Feature type	Aerated water (%)	Alcohol (%)	Total beverage bottles	Total feature artefacts
7	1788	1850	2 George St	Residential	Cellar		100.0%	79	457
6	1790	1830	100 George St	Residential	Pit		100.0%	4	96
2	1800	1860	15 Macquarie St	Residential	Dam		100.0%	15	2511
1	1820	1860	4 George St	Residential	Cesspit		100.0%	45	495
	1820	1860	Allotment 20 Church St	Baker's Arms/Star Inn	Rubbish Pit		100.0%	58	197
8	1830	1880	109 George St	Residential	Pit	5.1%	94.9%	39	248
6	1830	1890	100 George St	Residential	Well	15.8%	84.2%	57	1650
6	1861	1890	100 George St	Residential	Cesspit	11.1%	88.9%	9	512
6	1865	1890	100 George St	Residential	Cesspit	12.5%	87.5%	16	1137
3	1865	1895	45 Macquarie St	Residential	Well		100.0%	15	881
	1890	1917	Allotment 20 Church St	Star Inn	Cesspit	65.5%	34.5%	58	396
4	1890	1920	2 Taylor St	Residential	Cistern	17.4%	82.6%	27	307
5	1900	1935	13–15 Taylor St	Residential	Cistern	54.5%	45.5%	22	881

water supply and the growing social call for total alcohol abstinence were potentially key influences in increased consumption of aerated waters.

The nearby Hunt's Creek dam, constructed in 1853, provided a purer water supply to the town.[82] As Parramatta's waterways became polluted from the 1830s, archaeological evidence from the case-study sites suggests that some residents sought alternative sources of water by digging wells, and by the late 19th century, cisterns were common backyard features, as evidenced by three wells identified at case-study sites:

- An early settlement period well was located at 109 George Street (site 8). The date range for the well deposit artefacts is consistent with an early 19th-century to mid-19th-century occupation. While this property's well was not included as part of the case study, it is important to note because it contained no aerated water bottles.
- The Byrnes family occupied the property at 100 George Street (site 6) for all of Parramatta's "market town" period. A well was located in the side yard (adjacent Allotment 69) and, based on temporal data from this deposit, it was in use between 1830 and 1890. As Table 7.12 shows, aerated water bottles represent approximately 16 per cent of beverage bottles.
- Archaeological investigations found that the well at 45 Macquarie Street (site 3) was lined with the same type of bricks as used in the house construction and, therefore, was constructed at approximately the same time. Historical maps indicate that an outbuilding covered the well in the 1880s, suggesting it was abandoned at approximately that time. Yet dated artefacts recovered from the well suggest it was probably used for rubbish disposal until the 1890s. The contents of the well represent both "market town" and "feast and famine" periods of Parramatta's development. Despite the increased availability of aerated waters and the ever-increasing temperance pressures, no aerated water bottles were recovered.

Rubbish-filled cisterns, located in the backyards of two semidetached dwellings on Taylor Street (sites 4–5), contained "feast and famine" period artefacts, which indicate that freshwater issues continued into the 20th century. The dated artefacts in the deposits suggest that both cisterns were backfilled with rubbish once water supply was available in the town. These deposits produced the highest relative frequencies of aerated water bottles.

The evidence of government initiatives and private property efforts indicate that Parramatta's clean freshwater issues at the time were, to some extent, alleviated. Consequently, the increase of aerated water consumption was most likely not the result of clean water issues. Furthermore, the aerated water industry's rapid growth was not unique to Parramatta and is evidenced in towns and cities throughout New South Wales. There were ten aerated water firms in Sydney during the 1820s; by the 1920s, more than 500 aerated water firms had been established in Sydney and surrounding suburbs.[83] Residential assemblages from Sydney archaeological sites also show a pattern of increased aerated water consumption during the 19th century, but not as significant as in Parramatta. For example, dated residential cesspit deposits from the 710–722 George Street, Sydney archaeological investigation show no aerated waters from the early to mid-19th-century deposits, and only 2 per cent of the beverage bottles from the 1850–1900 deposits are aerated waters.[84] Furthermore, in the mid-19th-century abandoned wells at Clarence and Kent streets (mixed commercial and residential, 1840–1860) aerated water bottles represent less than 5 per cent of beverage bottles.[85]

The public consumption patterns for aerated waters are also evidenced in other archaeological collections from regional inns and hotels. In the cesspit (1830–1880) behind the Woolpack Inn at Old Marulan, south of Sydney on the Hume Highway near Goulburn, aerated waters represent 16 per cent of beverage bottles.[86] At the Red Cow Inn in nearby Penrith, New South Wales, 25 per cent of all artefacts (not only beverage bottles) recovered from late 19th-century deposits are aerated water bottles.[87] These results collectively demonstrate a change in public beverage consumption patterns to include aerated waters as an acceptable alternative to alcohol.

A more influential factor for the increased consumption of non-alcoholic beverages was the increased social influences of temperance movements. The consumption of aerated water and soft drinks, sometimes referred to as "temperance waters", was strongly encouraged by temperance reformers as an alternative to alcoholic consumption.[88] This comparative study suggests that changing social attitudes influenced a shift away from public consumption of alcohol and towards the drinking of aerated waters. Furthermore, it demonstrates variability in private (in-home) consumption.

One must consider that there were probably different patterns of non-alcoholic beverage consumption between public settings and homes. Much like modern times, a person visiting a public house may have been more likely to order a bottled beverage than to drink water. Conversely, drinking water at home may have been preferred. Yet despite these differences, there was a demonstrated increase in in-home consumption of aerated waters. Compared to the similarity to consumption patterns in

---

82 Larcombe 1973, 204–5.
83 D. Jones 2009.
84 Harris 2010.
85 Harris 2016.
86 Harris 2007.
87 Carney 1996, 8.
88 Blocker, Fahey and Tyrrell 2003, 570.

archaeological assemblages outside of Parramatta, clean water was probably not the main factor influencing the change, but rather the social influence of the temperance movements.

Discussion

Much of what is known of alcohol's role in the colony is from the public perspective. The popularity of 19th-century pubs, hotels and clubs demonstrates the social aspect of alcohol consumption that is still prevalent in the modern Australian culture, but little is known about 19th-century in-home drinking habits. Determining how public compares to private consumption patterns involves identification of in-home alcohol consumption patterns. An initial study of statistics from the archaeological record and historical records was conducted to accomplish this comparison. While historical documents record only imported alcohol, the catalogue of archaeological remains reflects both imported alcohol and those from the colonial beer and wine industry. Results of this comparison indicate that home-based beer and wine consumption was greater than historical records specify. This difference is likely due to the lack of statistics for the production of local colonial beer. Alternatively, bottle reuse practices may contribute to the statistical differences between these two studies. Spirits were imported in both bottles and casks, but import records only record the volume (that is, gallons) and not the container. Given the absence of glass manufacturers in the colony, spirits arriving in casks were bottled locally in any available (reusable) alcohol bottle form. Since beer and wine bottle types are the most common of these forms found in Parramatta's archaeological record, bottle reuse for spirits is a strong possibility. In either case, both historical statistics and the findings of this study indicate a preference for beer and wine over spirits.

Parramatta's public consumption of aerated waters is demonstrated with its popularity in social settings. Aerated waters were offered at social events, like the 1888 Parramatta District Liedertafel (singing group) concert that served aerated waters along with beer and spirits.[89] Aerated waters were also a popular beverage in late 19th-century pubs and hotels. This pattern of increased consumption of aerated waters is also observed for in-home consumption in Parramatta during the last half of the 19th century, but it did not yet equal the relative frequency of public consumption found in hotel assemblages. It was not until the early 20th century that the relative frequency of aerated waters equalled (or surpassed) in-home consumption of alcoholic beverages.

Schnapps has an interesting position in the 19th-century archaeological record. Nineteenth-century medical organisations denounced Udolpho Wolfe's advertising as deceptive.[90] Evidence of Wolfe's successful marketing campaign is preserved in the archives of Australian newspapers. While acknowledging its alcoholic content, many modern-day archaeologists tend to classify Udolpho Wolfe's Aromatic Schnapps as a patent medicine.[91] A few Australian archaeologists have discussed the link between patent medicines with high alcohol content and the population's desire for the appearance of respectability. Briggs' thesis on working-class respectability in Adelaide discusses the use of schnapps as medicine, but at the same time suggests its medicinal classification was a marketing ploy to maintain the illusion of respectability.[92] Lydon's article on a female-owned 19th-century boarding house in Sydney's Rocks neighbourhood suggests that alcohol- and opiate-based patent medicines afforded women a private and socially respectable means of alcohol consumption, however, there is no specific mention of schnapps.[93] Terry's article on a late 19th-century Queensland pastoral family includes an exemplary account of an ideal middle-class family whose artefact assemblage included only a few alcohol bottles and no identified opiate- or alcohol-based patent medicines.[94] Quirk's 2008 article on re-evaluating Victoria's goldfield towns is one of only a few archaeological studies discussing the possible connection between schnapps consumption and the temperance movement.[95]

Analysis results of the Parramatta study show increased popularity of schnapps during the second half of the 19th century. This consumption pattern is consistent with a population seeking a socially acceptable medical alternative to spirits while appearing to adhere to middle-class temperance values. Given the exponential growth of the temperance movement from the 1830s and Wolfe's genius for marketing, it is probably no coincidence that residents of Parramatta embraced schnapps as a socially acceptable source of alcohol.

Where schnapps may have been consumed under the guise of medicine to maintain respectability, aerated water consumption may represent an alternative to alcohol consumption. Advancements in bottling technology made aerated waters a more viable commodity, however, increased availability is not the only reason for their increased popularity during the 19th century. Contaminated water supply is one possibility but given the discussion above, and the colony-wide popularity of aerated waters in the second half of the 19th century, their popularity is more likely linked to abstinence from alcohol consumption.

---

89 *Cumberland Mercury* 16 June 1888, 6.
90 Hubbard 1853, 288.
91 Bonasera 2001; Harris et al. 2004, 42; Lun 2015, 22–3.
92 Briggs 2006, 109.
93 Lydon 1993, 37.
94 Terry 2013.
95 Quirk 2008.

Tobacco use – health, temperance and social values

Tobacco consumption was as much a part of the colonial culture as alcohol consumption. What is known about colonial tobacco consumption (in pipes) for much of the early 19th century comes from documentation of penal rations. During the convict era (1788–1868), convict workers were typically supplied with tobacco, usually 2 ounces (oz) per week, which was 104 oz annually and by the early 20th century, jailed prisoners received a 3 oz ration per week.[96]

In the 21st century, tobacco use's detrimental health effects are widely recognised. However, little was known of the cardiovascular disease, respiratory illnesses and cancers associated with tobacco use in the 19th century. Continuing the medical practices developed in the 16th century, tobacco use was seen to be widely beneficial as a cure for several different ailments, including toothaches, worms and lockjaw.[97] Furthermore, it calmed the nerves. It promoted concentration and quiet contemplation.[98] These perceptions continued throughout the 17th century, with tobacco smoking a prescribed remedy for many respiratory ailments. Lung cancer was rare in the 19th century because pipe and cigar smokers rarely inhaled, and cigarette smoking did not become commonplace until World War I.[99] Lip cancer was linked to pipe smokers in the 1820s, and by the mid-19th century, a growing number of anti-tobacco medical practitioners recognised the link between smoking and lung cancer.[100]

While the 19th-century medical community began to investigate the link between tobacco use and a growing list of ailments, the middle-class social convention of cleanliness (avoiding the smell) was probably more responsible for repressing tobacco smoking. Social conventions were established around public smoking for middle-class males and excluded middle-class women from indulging in any smoking activity. Under no circumstances was pipe smoking acceptable in public or social settings. While a middle-class Englishman would never smoke on the streets, this social convention was not strictly adhered to in the colony, however, smoking on the street in the company of a "lady" was an insult and any man was compelled to remove his cigar or pipe from his mouth before greeting a woman on the street.[101] Gentlemen had separate rooms in public establishments for smoking pipes and cigars, and, for home entertaining, gentlemen retired to another room to indulge their habits.[102] Cost was also a factor in tobacco use by social classes. Cigars and snuff were more expensive than pipe tobacco and thus more commonly used by more affluent members of society.

For working-class men and women, smoking was the norm, and it is estimated that as much as 80 per cent of working-class men indulged in pipe smoking. Working-class women also smoked, but, even among the working-class, public smoking was not condoned; women who did smoke in public were thought to be of low moral standing, yet almost all convicts (of both genders) used tobacco.[103] Smoking was discouraged in public and commercial facilities. There are accounts of men sitting and smoking their pipes outside the doors of hotels, inns, and pubs.[104] There was even a government inquiry into the abuse of smoking in railway workshops, but testimony by shop foremen stated that workers limited their smoking to the lavatories as the smoke served to mask the facility's stench.[105]

Temperance

Despite the efforts of social reformers, in particular temperance movements, to deride tobacco use, by some accounts, smoking in the colony steadily increased through the course of the 19th century.[106] In the mid-1830s negative articles on pipe and cigar smoking began appearing in Sydney's newspapers.[107] By the early 1840s, such articles expanded to link smoking with alcohol abuse, with such statements as:

> Smoking and chewing tobacco led to drinking, drinking to transportation, and transportation, very often, to premature death.[108]

> … smoking is the great inlet to drunkenness, because when people smoke they spit, and when they spit, their blood is thickened, and when that is the case they feel thirsty; ergo, they must needs go to the alehouse and get drunk.[109]

There were several articles in the media expressing public indignation regarding the linking of the two habits.[110]

Archaeological evidence

Of the four main forms of tobacco use during the 19th century (pipes, cigars, snuff and cigarettes), pipe-smoking provides the most tangible evidence. Clay tobacco pipes are durable artefacts, even though they had a short three-week life expectancy and were casually discarded. Cigars and snuff have poor representation in the archaeological

---

96 Walker 1984, 11.
97 Loddenkemper and Kreuter 2015, 9.
98 Tyrrell 2008, 2.
99 Walker 1980, 394.
100 Walker 1980, 395.
101 Walker 1984, 32.
102 People's Publishing Company 1885, 157–8.
103 Walker 1984, 11.
104 Walker 1984, 32.
105 Blainey 2003, 315–16.
106 Blainey 2003, 322.
107 Harris 2021, 194–7.
108 *Sydney Herald* 28 March 1836, 2.
109 *Sydney Herald* 8 January 1840, 2.
110 *Sydney Gazette and New South Wales Advertiser* 2 November 1841, 3; *Sydney Herald* 8 January 1841, 2; *Sydney Monitor*, 25 October 1834, 2; *Temperance Advocate and Australasian Commercial and Agricultural Intelligencer* 20 January 1841, 5.

record. Their associated paraphernalia (mouthpieces, cigar cutters, snuff boxes) are rare. Equally rare in 19th-century collections is evidence of cigarettes. Cigarettes were first introduced during the Crimean War (1853–1856) but did not become a common form of tobacco consumption until World War I,[111] which is beyond the end of the case-study time period.

Davies' and Gojak and Stuart's articles contend that analysis of tobacco pipes has the potential for understanding social, economic and political aspects of colonial Australia.[112] Furthermore, tobacco pipe analysis contributes insights into health consequences and social constraints of tobacco use in 19th-century colonial Parramatta society.

Clay tobacco pipes have been the subject of numerous archaeological studies, but only a few have addressed the connection between pipe smoking and Victorian values. Reckner and Brighton's article on working-class vices in 19th-century New York's Five Points discusses the increasing awareness of health issues related to smoking and discusses the link between tobacco and respectability.[113] In Australia, in Briggs' study of working-class respectability in Port Adelaide, she "developed a model for assessing the integration of the ideology of respectability into working-class lives". She groups all aspects of social reform values under the umbrella of respectability.[114] Briggs' theory is not adhered to for this research because of its one-dimensional interpretation of these values as having a goal of respectability through self-reliance. Briggs fails to examine the intricate composition of the social structure that recognised or embraced these individual values; instead, she considers respectability as a single value. Fortunately, the study does include a useful analysis of tobacco use in working-class homes that demonstrates a varying range of attitudes.

The analysis of tobacco use conducted in the Parramatta study is twofold. The initial analysis for tobacco pipes is a chronological assessment to determine if patterns identified in the analysis results may be related to tobacco sourcing during early colonial times. Subsequently, consideration is given to the social class of households, and how analysis results may indicate how social standing or temperance reformation influenced tobacco-use patterns.

Table 7.13 shows there was a lower relative frequency of tobacco pipes (3.9 per cent) in the convict-settlement times (c. 1790–1830). This probably relates to the uncertain supply of tobacco during the 1790s that drove up the imported tobacco price to 10–15 shillings per pound. Also, during this time, there was a government prohibition on colonial cultivation of tobacco because all arable land was needed for food crops. When this ban was lifted in the early 1800s, the colonial supply market was slow developing, because at that time no one in the colony knew the proper procedures for tobacco cultivation.[115] With the ban lifted, the price of imported tobacco dropped to 8 shillings per pound and gradually continued to drop over the next ten years to reach a low of 2 shillings 6 pence per pound to compete with the increasing domestic market.[116] During this time (between 1820 and 1850), the relative frequency of tobacco pipes in the Parramatta case study rose. For two of the three sites dated to this period, the relative frequencies rose to 3.7 and 4.4 per cent. At site 2, the higher relative frequency of tobacco pipes (19.35 per cent) suggests the habit of smoking was a constant activity. Results of artefact analysis from the dam deposits suggest they represent a mix of pre-residential land clearance, agricultural activities and the site's post-1830s residential occupation. As pipe-smoking is a common activity associated with labour, the high relative frequency of tobacco pipes may be influenced by land clearance and agricultural activities associated with this allotment and the adjacent field.[117]

In 1822, government policy changed again with Governor Brisbane going beyond allowing tobacco cultivation to encouraging domestic cultivation, and ultimately to establishing government-owned tobacco fields at Port Macquarie's convict settlement. The price of imported tobacco rose back up to 3 shillings per pound by 1824, and advertising for colonial tobacco states that the quality was equal to foreign and sold at a reduced price. Advertisements for colonial tobacco stated it was sold by the barrel and no specific price was listed. The government sold a total of 30,946 lbs of domestically grown tobacco in 1824.[118] The ready supply of domestic tobacco may account, in part, for the spike in the relative frequency of tobacco pipes recovered from the fill deposits in the dam (pond) at 15 Macquarie Street (site 2).

Drought in 1826–1827 caused a drop in colonial tobacco supply in the 1830s, which may account for the drop in tobacco pipes' relative frequencies evidenced in the 4 George Street deposit (4.44 per cent). The colonial tobacco industry survived the drought and eventually grew through the efforts of private sector growers. After that, the growth of the industry and the supply of colonial and imported tobacco was, for the most part, stable.

From the 1830s, other factors began to influence tobacco consumption. For a decade, the medical community had been making links between smoking and ill health, temperance reformers began linking smoking with alcohol abuse, and middle-class social etiquette tried to dissuade people from smoking through a series of limiting social conventions. For Parramatta, the effects of medical and social reform efforts are reflected in

---

111 Walker 1984, 4, 13.
112 Davies 2011; Gojak and Stuart 1999.
113 Reckner and Brighton 1999.
114 Briggs 2006.

115 *Sydney Gazette and New South Wales Advertiser* 22 January 1804, 4.
116 *Sydney Gazette and New South Wales Advertiser* 4 August 1810, 2.
117 Casey & Lowe 2012, vol. 3, 108.
118 Walker 1984, 10.

7 The archaeology of personal health and social reforms

Table 7.13 Relative frequencies calculated for tobacco pipes from case-study sites in chronological order.

Site Number	Address	Social class status	Date range	Feature type	Minimum Item Count	%	Feature total
6	100 George St	Working	1790–1830	Rubbish pit	3	3.13	96
7	2 George St	Working	1810–40s	Cellar	17	3.72	457
8	109 George St	Middle/gentry	1820–60	Rubbish pit	2	0.81	248
2	15 Macquarie St	Working	1823–41	Dam	486	19.35	2511
1	4 George St	Middle	1820–60	Cesspit (6024)	22	4.44	495
3	45 Macquarie St	Middle	1860–90	Well	4	0.45	881
6	100 George St	Middle/gentry	1865–90	Cesspit (2370)	2	0.58	345
6	100 George St	Middle/gentry	1865–1930	Cesspit (2369)	7	0.62	1137
6	100 George St	Middle/gentry	1865–1940	Cesspit (2206)	5	0.96	521
4	2 Taylor St	Middle	1890–1920	Cistern	0	0	307
5	13–15 Taylor St	Middle	1900–30	Cistern	0	0	268

the archaeological record, with a steady decline in the relative frequencies of tobacco pipes from the mid-19th century and a total absence of tobacco pipes from the late 19th-century to early 20th-century deposits.

Discussion

The assessment of in-home tobacco use is limited to analysis of tobacco pipe use. Any attempts at a comparative analysis of the changing methods of tobacco consumption during the 19th century are beyond this study's scope, as cigars, snuff and cigarettes leave little in the archaeological record. While analysis included more than 52,000 artefacts, the only other tobacco-related artefact identified is a cigarette tobacco tin from the early 20th-century cistern at 13–15 Taylor Street.

What was required for the assessment of tobacco pipe-smoking practices in Parramatta was a dichotomous analytical approach, distinguishing between two significant influences on 19th-century tobacco pipe smoking. In early colonial times, supply was a major factor; once the tobacco supply was stable in the 1830s, science and social reform influenced tobacco smoking in pipes. The analysis results are consistent with historical documentation. Results for the early colonial deposits (1790–1820s) conform to the datable fluctuation patterns in tobacco supply. About the same time as the stabilisation of the tobacco supply was achieved, social conventions began to restrict smoking patterns. Also, temperance movements began campaigning for smoking abstinence. These two initiatives influenced the decline in tobacco pipe smoking evidenced in post-1830 deposits to the point of total absence by the 20th century.

Personal health is comprised of the proactive and reactive attitudes to wellness on an individual basis. Personal health is considered in three basic categories: proactive and reactive health care; hygiene and grooming; and vices. Archaeological evidence of these groups is found in a site's material culture. Artefacts associated with an individual's choices in healthcare treatment are consultation with orthodox medical practitioners, alternative medical practitioners or self-medication, and the selection of one over the other depends on a number of factors, including economic status, access to professional medical practitioners and personal preferences. Hygiene and grooming-related artefacts demonstrate in part the individual's or household's aspirations to adhere to cleanliness habits that are associated with respectability. Vices that are detrimental to good health are highly influenced by social reform values, and the artefacts, such as alcohol bottles and tobacco pipes, indicate the level to which these values influence individuals and households.

Chapter 8
COLONIAL PARRAMATTA: A MEDICAL ANTHROPOLOGICAL APPROACH TO HEALTH AND CLASS

Victorian values influenced approaches to health by promoting cleanliness in 19th-century Australian culture. The previous chapters provide a cohesive discussion that connects historical, archaeological, medical and sociological evidence within the framework of medical anthropology to examine social conventions and their influence on health in 19th-century Parramatta. The assertion is that cleanliness of the body (internal and external) and soul fostered good health. A case study is used to interpret archaeological data from Parramatta to determine how the archaeological record can contribute to this argument alongside other disciplines.

This research centres around a series of basic inquiries designed to examine the evidence for clarification of the impact cultural values had on cleanliness and health. Addressing these questions essentially requires an analytical structure that results in a measured, theoretical approach. Brown and Closser contend that medical anthropology concepts and methods draw from all aspects of anthropology to understand broad social and cultural contexts.[1] Furthermore, Witeska-Mlynarczyk emphasises the utility of medical anthropology in multidisciplinary research.[2] Therefore, my theoretical approach has incorporated several disciplines under the aegis of a medical anthropology framework. The interdisciplinary nature of this research led to the formulation of a research design that focuses on class structure, health concerns and approaches to health treatment. The following analysis discusses the interpretation of the findings.

Within this anthropological framework, consideration is given to Benedict's contention that, to understand one trait of culture, there must be an understanding of the culture as a whole,[3] wherein understanding attitudes towards health in Australian culture necessitates comprehension of its cultural heritage and development. Rosecrance's characterisation of Australian culture provided a background for Australia's cultural development and served as a foundation for assessing social change in colonial New South Wales.[4] While the background research encompasses all of New South Wales, Parramatta's location on the edge of the frontier provided a specific and more focused view of colonial cultural development, history and archaeology in this remote settlement.

Inspired by Zierden and Reitz's 2016 work in Charleston, South Carolina, the selection of case-study sites was made to provide a city-wide perspective of class over the 19th century.[5] The application of post-processual approaches in the analysis of artefact collections is crucial to this argument, because it allows for interpretation without being influenced by narrowly materialist preconceived patterns. Furthermore, the selection of case-study sites, features and artefact collections uses Schiffer's theoretical framework for the analysis of collections from sealed contexts.[6]

Understanding the impact of Victorian values first necessitates answering the question "Did Victorian values dominate the colonial social system?" and the answer to this question requires an understanding of class formation. As previously discussed, Marx defines class in terms of exploitation and dominance, and Young contends that labour is the fundamental defining factor that separates the classes.[7] If labour is the basic factor of class, then power is how one class gains dominance over another. Settled as a penal colony, the cultural fragmentation experienced in early New South Wales and the absence of aristocracy resulted in the labouring classes attaining a more prominent role. The emerging colonial classes were based on capital, and land was the principal capital in the New South Wales colony. Aspirations of the labouring class to acquire land allowed squatters to achieve that all-important first step towards emulating their homeland's landed gentry. Emulating the perceived social conventions of the gentry furthered their attempt to elevate themselves to those standards. It could be proposed that these pastoralists were central to forming the middle class in the colony. During the colony's formative years, the middle class represented a minority of the population, yet they were major employers of the predominant labouring class that consisted of convicts, emancipists and expirees. With dominance or power or both over their workers, the middle class was able to influence the workers' social values. While Beaudry and colleagues' contention that the working class had the ability to formulate its own social values, and despite Abercrombie and Turner's assertions that subordinate classes do not necessarily embrace the ideology of the dominant class, for 19th-century Parramatta, Victorian

---

1 P.J. Brown and Closser 2016.
2 Witeska-Mlynarczyk 2012.
3 Benedict 1934.
4 Rosecrance 1964.
5 Zierden and Reitz 2016.
6 Schiffer 1987.
7 E.O. Wright 2015, xi; Young 1988, 5.

values had a dominant influence on the colonial social system.[8]

Next, a definition of Victorian values is required to support the contention that health was the overarching theme of these values.[9] Conversely, most historical archaeologists collectively group these values as lifestyle choices to emulate "respectability" without regard for the actions of reform used as the vehicles to promote compliance.[10] This volume of research demonstrates that these social conventions are a compilation of factors from many disciplines to explain how Victorian values, operating within the colonial culture, promoted a healthy lifestyle.

Parramatta's location on the frontier of colonial expansion allows a case study that examines its response to Victorian values of respectability (personal hygiene and grooming, sobriety, piety, work ethic and chastity) and contributes to the understanding of the effectiveness of reform efforts on health in the whole colony. These reforms are demonstrated in both the historical and archaeological records. Applying this broader perspective to the archaeological record requires a dichotomous approach to enable the independent examination of environmental reforms and social reforms that promoted clean lifestyle practices that affected the health practices of Parramatta residents during the long 19th century.

Environmental reforms are beneficial initiatives for the collective wellbeing of the settlement. These reforms are further subdivided into public and private health initiatives. Public health initiatives consisted of government reforms to control or eradicate contagious diseases on a colonial basis, while local initiatives in Parramatta improved the infrastructure, such as drains and water supply, and were undertaken by government schemes and individual landowners. Social reforms support the health of individuals through modification of clean lifestyle behaviour patterns. Personal health is a multifaceted topic comprised of themes relating to medicine, nutrition, hygiene, social class and colonial convictism. Using a city-wide approach allows for exploring the transition from traditional to orthodox health care throughout the periods of Parramatta's development.[11] These reforms are organised within the framework of the four themes that emerged during the research process. Presented individually, these themes argue the impact of Victorian values on health through cleanliness in the setting of colonial Parramatta:

- Cleanliness was the thread that connected health to Victorian values.
- Victorian values supported the advancement of orthodox medicine.
- There were public and private faces of compliance with Victorian values.
- There was evidence of discrimination against the lower classes that prevented the working class from raising its social status.

The following discussions of these four themes explain how Victorian values influenced the health of colonial Parramatta.

Cleanliness is next to godliness: a primary indicator of respectability and compliance with Victorian values

Cleanliness has been an essential component of social values since the 18th century.[12] Woven throughout this research is the recurring theme of cleanliness and the argument that cleanliness is synonymous with health. A clean environment, body and soul reflects a healthy environment and, as Smith contends,[13] this thread of body, soul and health connects all aspects of Victorian values.

Environmental reforms for cleanliness

Public environmental reforms took two forms: the New South Wales government initiatives to control or eradicate contagious diseases through vaccinations and quarantine, and sanitation initiatives for improvement to the infrastructure needed to ensure Parramatta's residents lived in clean, mould-free homes and had access to fresh water. History has taught that, if properly followed, preventative regimes rather than the cure of disease have a more significant impact on health.[14] In New South Wales, adopting vaccination procedures for contagious diseases in 1828 was much earlier than many other countries. In the absence of vaccination, the government was motivated to pass quarantine legislation to ensure the population remained clean of epidemics and contagions.[15]

Attitudes towards cleanliness in hospital environments changed significantly during the 19th century. While the extensive archaeological investigations conducted at the site of all Parramatta's hospitals detailed their structural remains, they lacked the historical narrative to address these facilities' hygienic conditions.[16] Data on sanitary conditions in these facilities are found in historical records and independent historians' scholarly research. The earliest Parramatta hospital (1789) consisted of one ward, where there was a serious potential for spreading contagious disease. Overcrowding and the single-ward situation continued in the second hospital (1794) and the only improvement to the 1818 Colonial Hospital was the addition of verandahs all around for better ventilation.

---

8 Abercrombie and Turner 1978, 150; Beaudry, Cook and Mrozowski 1991, 279.
9 Haley 1979, 3.
10 Harris 2021, 159.
11 Evans 1983; Hagger 1979; Lewis 2014.

12 Porter 1982, 326.
13 V. Smith 2007.
14 Bynum 1994, 55; Foley 1995, 10.
15 Jamison 1804, 2; New South Wales Health Department 1997, 61.
16 Casey 2005; Casey & Lowe 2005b.

The first segregation of patients happened in 1848 but this separation entailed using the upper floor to house the "unclean" paupers; no consideration was given to isolating potentially contagious patients. The acceptance of Lister's germ theory led to resident surgeon George Pringle's 1867 introduction of antiseptic medical practices at the hospital, and, by the late 19th century, separation of the contagious patients was finally achieved by a ward contained in a separate purpose-built facility.

Influential studies on sanitation reform helped Parramatta's regional government to develop schemes to ensure a clean and healthy living environment.[17] Initiatives such as the "town drain" helped to alleviate unhealthy mildew and mould within low-lying dwellings.[18] However, the government's failure to improve drainage in a timely fashion left the landowners to deal with this issue as best they could during Parramatta's first 30 years. Landowner initiatives evidenced during archaeological excavations for three low-lying properties in the case study ranged from simple channels to nearby streams or constructed dams, to more elaborate interconnected drainage systems for more severe drainage issues. Properties located on an alluvial terrace or slope with sandy soil had adequate natural drainage, as did the late-19th-century developments of properties located on elevated land that had municipal storm drainage.

The rapidly expanding population, growing number of government institutions and Parramatta's commercial and industrial development compromised the town's water supply with organic waste and toxins contaminating drinking, bathing and laundry water. Under the auspices of several New South Wales governors, early government initiatives made inroads to solving the problem. Two existing archaeological sites are government-constructed freshwater dams: the 1818 "town dam" (the Marsden Street Weir) spans the Parramatta River at approximately the point where the salt water meets the fresh water, and the 1850s Hunts Creek Dam two kilometres north of central Parramatta. Eventually, this issue became the onus of a reluctant local government; due to either a lack of funds or poor planning, it took nearly 60 years to complete a freshwater supply scheme.

In the interim, landowners were left to deal with obtaining clean, fresh water individually. Whether for convenience or by necessity, a clean water supply was achieved by either sinking wells, installing cisterns or paying to have clean water carted in. The structural remains of wells and cisterns, identified during archaeological investigations at seven of the eight case-study sites, denote a change in residential sourcing of fresh water from wells to cisterns towards the end of the 19th century.

Bathing was both a preventative and reactionary measure against disease. Many physicians considered it a medicinal stimulant.[19] If bathing was the social benchmark for cleanliness and the river was polluted, the question remains: where did the most people bathe? While the promotion of cleanliness and health through ablutions is a social reform, the needed fresh water required environmental reform. The 1886 *Parramatta Public Baths Act* provided for the construction of the riverside Centennial Baths in 1888. Unfortunately, no archaeological evidence of these baths remains due to 20th-century redevelopment.[20] The archaeological artefact collections do provide insight into the accoutrements for bathing (basins and ewers), such as those found in most case-study artefact collections. These artefacts indicate in-home ablutions but also show that it was limited to sponge baths (Table 7.7). No evidence of bathtubs used for full-body bathing was found during archaeological investigations at case-study sites.

Clean clothing, another outward marker of cleanliness and health, required fresh or unpolluted water because fabric washed in polluted water potentially transferred infectious diseases from fabric to skin. Whether convict, working class or middle class, all individuals strove to maintain the appearance of cleanliness by their attire. Most of what is known of laundry activities comes from Parramatta's historical record, including the convict laundry facilities at the Parramatta Female Factory (Figure 8.1) and advertisements by commercial establishments for laundresses.[21] For case-study sites, the historical research indicates laundry structures were located at working-class, middle-class and middle-class gentry sites (sites 2, 3 and 6). None was explicitly located or identified during archaeological excavations. Historical scholarship indicates that all classes of society recognised the importance of clean clothing. Yet it is uncertain if individuals' compliance with this social value was for social acceptance or for health purposes, or both.

Social reforms

Social reforms forge a strong connection between cleanliness and health. There is more to cleanliness than bathing and clean clothes. Personal hygiene and grooming practices also promote health and cleanliness. One personal hygiene practice in particular, good oral hygiene, is vital in maintaining good health. The mouth is the first step in the digestive system, breaking down food into nutritional components for nutrient absorption needed by the body for health and development. Mant and Roberts' archaeological study in 18th-century and 19th-century London presents an analysis that can be applied to the colony's mainly English, Irish and Scottish settlers. It links increased rates of dental decay with changes to dietary patterns that consisted mostly of an

---

17 Peterson 1979, 86.
18 Dusting 2016; 2017; Higginbotham 1981.
19 Jackson 2014, 136.
20 Casey & Lowe 2014.
21 *Sydney Gazette and New South Wales Advertiser* 13 March 1827, 1.

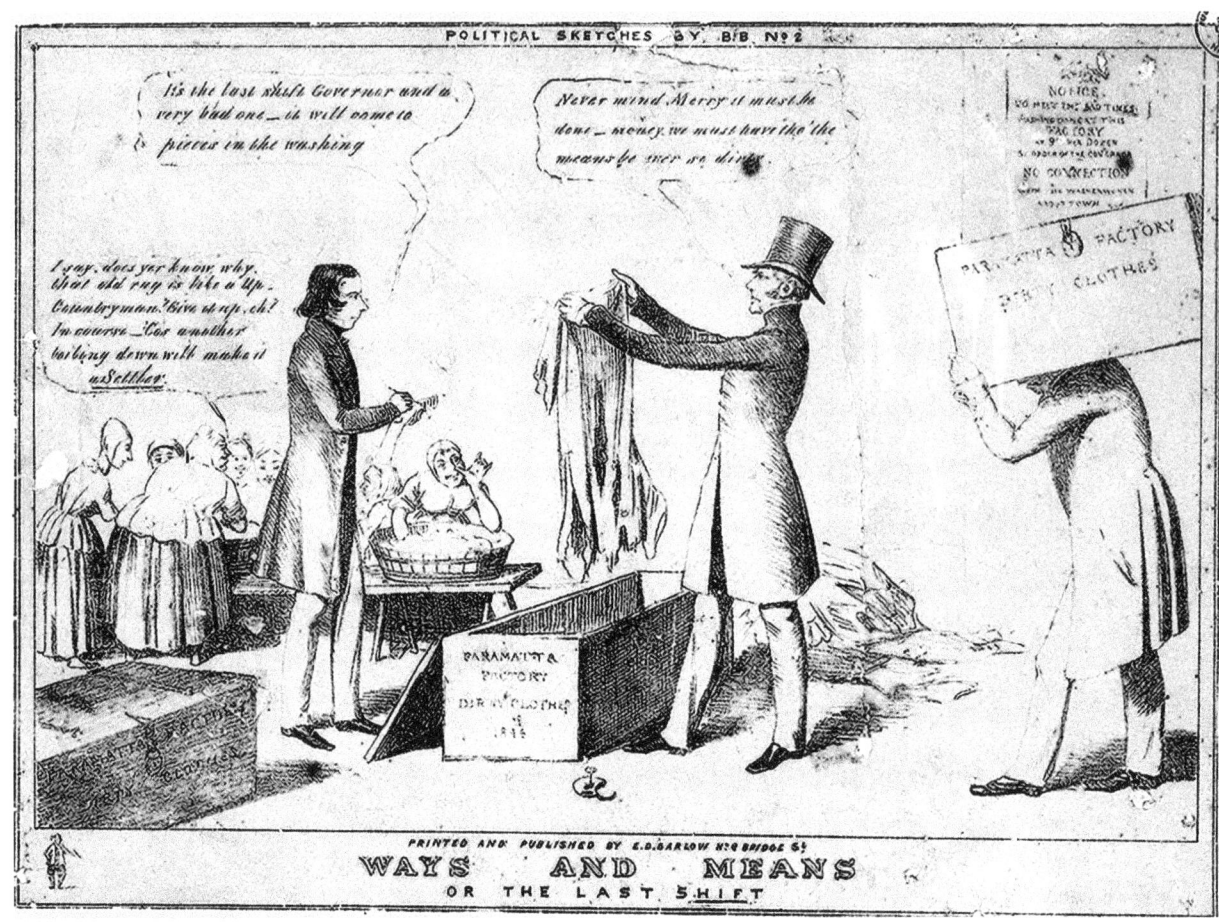

Figure 8.1 An 1844 sketch of female convicts doing laundry at the Parramatta Female Factory. Source: State Library of New South Wales (a2255004/DL PXX 66).

increase in carbohydrates and the introduction of refined sugars.[22] As author Jane Austen's personal letters reveal, this increase in caries was noticeable in the middle and upper classes of British society, the two socio-economic classes that could afford the costly foods associated with these changes in dietary patterns.[23]

Artefactual evidence contributed to class-specific use-pattern analysis for oral hygiene practices. There were two available methods for teeth cleaning during the case-study periods: biodegradable chalk and twigs, and more durable bone toothbrushes and tooth powder or paste pots. Associated material culture available during Parramatta's "early" and "convict settlement" periods was mostly organic materials that are not often distinguished in an archaeological context. The more durable items (toothbrushes and pots) became increasingly available by the mid-19th century. A class-related analysis of oral hygiene items at first examination indicated only middle-class and middle-class gentry households practised good oral hygiene. This result does not consider the limited availability of durable toothcare items during early settlement, when most case-study households were

working class. Also, there is the possibility that working-class households did not embrace the new modalities for preventative care for oral hygiene and thus their oral hygiene was poor.

Grooming is principally an outward expression of cleanliness. Along with bodily cleanliness and clean clothing, appearance portrayed by good hygiene was an affectation of respectability. Public hygiene is a collection of habits and customs that are insignificant when taken individually but observed collectively promote health and convey a perceived sense of compliance with prevailing social values. Artefact collections from the case-study sites contained a variety of grooming items. All case-study artefact collections included fragrance bottles. While fragrances are used for many purposes, such as enhancing moods and relieving stress, they were historically most likely used to mask unpleasant body odours. Artefact collections from the the late 19th-century (1870s–1900s) case-study sites (sites 4 and 5), are middle-class households and contain shaving accessories, which are consistent with changing late-19th-century clean-shaven fashion for facial hair.

Cleanliness is more than an individual's outward hygiene practices; it is also the cleanliness of the body's interior. What a person puts in their body is a sign of

---

22 Mant and Roberts 2014.
23 Woolsey 1908, 200.

cleanliness and at the same time promotes good health. What an individual eats and drinks, as well as illnesses and medication, affect their health and wellness. For most Christian denominations, doctrines promote both physical and spiritual cleanliness. The Christian sacrament of baptism is a symbolic cleansing of the soul that has its origins in the Jewish purification ritual Tevilah.[24] Anglo-Christians sought spiritual salvation through clean living. The middle class assimilated this doctrine into its values, while, as a result of the widespread acceptance of germ theory, the 19th-century orthodox medical community was emphatic in its contention that both external and internal cleanliness was the single best preventative practice to promote health and wellbeing.

Vices and cleanliness

Substance abuse of alcohol and tobacco were vices regarded by temperance activists as unclean habits. Excessive drinking and smoking were considered signs of an unclean body and, therefore, an unhealthy body. As markers of disrespectability, the indulgence in these vices was evidenced in both the public and private arenas. Government control of alcohol consumption played a part in Australian culture even before the First Fleet landed on the shores of Botany Bay, with Lord Sydney's plan for an alcohol-free colony. After food, alcohol became one of the essential commodities in the colony due in part to the use of spirits as barter. So great was the market for spirits in the colony that, during the 19th century, the economic control of spirit licensing resulted in two significant historical events: the controversy over the ban of domestic distilleries that culminated with the Rum Rebellion, and Macquarie's importation exclusivity deal that financed the construction of Sydney's public hospital, popularly known as the "Rum Hospital".

The virtuous call by physical puritans for temperance in alcohol consumption became increasingly louder from the mid-19th century. Historian Matt Allen explains the success of alcohol temperance as the philanthropic elite enforcing their values on the behaviour of their social inferiors.[25] Temperance organisations received support from the churches. In colonial New South Wales many of the magistrates were clergymen, who could use their position to pass harsh sentences on individuals arrested for public drunkenness. Civic leaders, government officials and religious leaders all thought alcohol abuse was linked with disreputable behaviour. One small success for temperance movements was achieved when New South Wales Governor George Gipps (term 1838–1846), a supporter of temperance, halted the issuance of rum as part of the rations for imperial troops and increased the excise take on all spirits.[26] The medical profession linked alcohol consumption with physical ailments and insanity.

Although further study of this aspect is beyond this book's scope, the stresses of living in the new colony could have led to mental health issues, which was self-managed by excessive drinking, or these same stresses were drowned in alcohol that then led to a similar outcome. Either way, in 1856 the Select Committee for the Adelaide Lunatic Asylum stated it believed that drunkenness was more of a contributing factor to insanity than heredity.[27]

Due largely to this increasing influence of the temperance movements from the mid-19th century, drinking patterns began to change. The archaeological record suggests that the response to these movements was subjective, with some adopting a dichotomous pattern for alcohol consumption for public and private drinking practices. The comparative study of alcohol consumption for Parramatta public houses with private households follows the structuration theory, showing that, while aware of social rules, some residents manipulated these rules to their own purposes. There was a substantial decrease in public alcohol consumption during the second half of the 19th century in public houses, with increased consumption of aerated waters (Table 7.12). At the same time, the archaeological record demonstrates agency for in-home drinking patterns. Initially, the decline in alcohol consumption in private homes was far less than that of public houses. However, by the 1890s, an increased aerated water consumption pattern was apparent. Furthermore, from the 1860s, there was an increase in the in-home consumption of medicinal schnapps, which is more likely attributed to efforts to circumvent temperance standards than the medicinal benefits of schnapps.

Like alcohol, tobacco consumption was an integral part of colonial culture. In a thesis on the archaeology of working-class respectability in Adelaide, Briggs maintains smoking was a recreational pastime, describes attitudes towards smoking in terms of respectability and contends that middle-class temperance movements considered smoking sinful and wicked.[28] This interpretative approach to smoking habits and social respectability is typical in much of the archaeological scholarship. The studies emphasise the morality of temperance but fail to consider the deeper health reasons for refraining from smoking.[29] There were many reasons for smoking during the 19th century; recreation was just one reason. The narcotic nicotine in tobacco ultimately made its increased use a medical addiction more than a recreational pastime. Furthermore, the social ritual of sharing a pipe, or even smoking to mask the foul smells in the workplace and toilet blocks are just as apparent reasons. Additionally, archaeologists give little consideration to the adverse effects of smoking on health, or even recognition that many of the temperance advocates against smoking were medical practitioners

---

24 Jones 2001.
25 Allen 2013, 150.
26 Blocker, Fahey and Tyrrell 2003, 75.

27 Piddock 2007, 199.
28 Briggs 2006, 23.
29 Beaudry and Mrozowski 1988, 18; Davies 2011; Gojak and Stuart 1999; Tyrrell 2008, 1.

who were starting to link tobacco smoking to heart disease, respiratory illnesses and cancer. One exception to this mainstream archaeological approach is Reckner and Brighton's (1999) article on working-class vices in the 19th-century Five Points neighbourhood of New York City, which notes the health concerns related to the call for temperance of tobacco and alcohol in the workplace.

Unlike alcohol, little effort was made in New South Wales during the first half of the 19th century to limit systemic tobacco use. More than the economic, health or political aspects of tobacco use, anti-smoking social attitudes were related to its offensive smell in many social settings.[30] From the mid-19th century, recognition of medical ailments associated with smoking and efforts to curtail smoking were incorporated into the campaigns of organisations promoting alcohol temperance practices. The archaeological record for the case study indicates these medical and social reform efforts resulted in a steady decline in the relative frequencies of pipe-smoking from the mid-19th century to the late 19th century in Parramatta with a complete cessation of pipe-smoking, at least for the middle class, by the 20th century.

Attitudes towards medical reform

A common theme in Victorian literature, found in novels by Eliot and Dickens, is the condemning portrait of society's obsession with logic and scientific advancement at the expense of the imagination.[31] This theme applies to changing social attitudes towards the science of medicine. Medical history research demonstrates that the advancements in orthodox medicine supposedly allowed it to increase its dominance over traditional medicine. The shift from traditional to orthodox medicine was aided by government regulations intended to protect the population from malpractice by untrained and uncertified charlatans: for example, the 1876 *New South Wales Register of Druggists and Chemists*; *Medical Practitioners (Amendment) Act 1900* (Act No. 33, 1900). Other government regulations were public health initiatives to control and eradicate contagious diseases through vaccinations. The transition was further supported through social attitudes, such as those portrayed in Victorian literature. One way to see which medical approach dominated Parramatta is to look to the archaeological record for use patterns of proprietary and patent medicines (often of dubious efficiency) versus those of compounding chemists, who filled prescriptions written by orthodox medical practitioners. Unfortunately, the analysis that attempted to explore this issue was inconclusive due to product labelling methods.[32] During the first half of the 19th century, most chemists and patent medicine manufacturers used generic bottle forms with paper labelling, a practice that continued to some extent for the second half of the 19th century.

The science of medical reform

Numerous scientific advancements played a crucial role in 19th-century medicine, including germ theory, antiseptic medical practices and vaccinations for smallpox, cholera and typhoid. The Parramatta medical community played a vital role in bringing these advances to the colony. Most noticeable of these achievements were the 1804 program initiated by Assistant Surgeon John Savage to inoculate Parramatta children against smallpox, Surgeon George Pringle's introduction of antiseptic surgery to New South Wales in 1867 and Ellen Curling's 1876 establishment of the first medical practice in all of Australia that specialised in women's medicine.

One explanation for the rise in popularity of patent medicines in the colony was the lack of availability of and lack of access to traditional medicine from "wise women". This changing medication pattern was true for colonial New South Wales for two reasons. First, many convicts had originally come from rural origins where they had access to local healers, but had been transplanted into urban settings due to changing economic and work conditions. So, even before transport to the penal colony, they had already been forced to turn to other sources for their medicines. Second, new legislation in Britain and New South Wales precluded these healers from practising in traditional roles. The new orthodox medicine became the prerogative of the medical profession. Instead of incorporating traditional medicine into a comprehensive approach to medical treatment, the orthodox approach to medicine was to eradicate traditional medical approaches. Instead of educating traditional medical practitioners about germ theory and instructing them in the importance of cleanliness in preventing the spread of germs and disease, the orthodox community strove to eliminate them as a group. Much of this elimination process came with the support of government regulations. In 1876, chemists were required to be certified by the New South Wales Registry of Druggists. Barbers were banned from the practice of tooth extraction by the *New South Wales Dentistry Act* of 1900.

Noteworthy attitude changes that were prevalent during the 19th century were those concerned with women's health. The orthodox medical community's prejudicial attitude towards midwives was most damaging to the tradition of midwifery-assisted birthing in Australia. The hazards of childbirth were responsible for more deaths than epidemic diseases.[33] Prenatal infant deaths, such as those found during archaeological excavations on the grounds of the Parramatta Hospital, were common during early settlement. Advancements in orthodox obstetrics were seen to reduce this pattern. While some midwives in the colony were trained and certified in British institutions, such as the Ladies Medical College, women such as Ellen Curling (site 5) were officially banned from practice because the New South Wales

---

30 People's Publishing Company 1885, 280.
31 Rahn 2011, 1.
32 Harris 2019.

33 Cartwright 1972, 232.

Medical Board did not recognise their certification. The orthodox medical community fostered midwives' portrayal as being much like Mrs Gamp, who is an offensive caricature of a Victorian homecare nurse and midwife in Dickens' *Martin Chuzzlewit*. Her depiction as an unclean, drunken and ponderous character profoundly affected Australian attitudes towards this class of medical practitioners.[34]

The mid-19th century social acceptance of the scientific approach to medicine meant that the decline of the traditional midwife was inevitable. Proposed New South Wales legislation in 1895 and 1898 sought the registration of all midwifery nurses, but regulation for the registration of midwifery nurses was not achieved until 1924.[35] Ultimately, obstetric medicine could only be practised by certified physicians with the assistance of the new style of midwifery nurse. This new breed of midwife-nurse was trained in schools, such as Florence Nightingale's secular nursing school, to be a proficient assistant in all aspects of obstetrics.[36] The Parramatta Female Factory had closed in 1848 when the building was repurposed as a facility for invalid and lunatic prisoners.[37] This closure meant women previously accommodated in its lying-in hospital, which was serviced by midwives, subsequently sought the orthodox medical staff's services at the Parramatta Hospital.

Similarly, the orthodox medical community began to replace traditional remedies with more modern medicines. The opiate-based pain medicines of the orthodox practitioners supplanted the traditional remedies for toothaches (clove oil), muscle pain (mustard seed plasters), headaches (ginger and lavender) and many more ailments.[38] Opiate-based drugs are the most effective medicines to control pain and also treat symptoms of other ailments such as congestion and coughs, but they come with side effects. Besides being addictive, opiate-based medicines often cause nausea and constipation. In artefact collections from case-study sites, laxative bottles were recovered from two middle-class households (45 Macquarie Street and the Wentworth Estates) and one middle-class gentry household deposit (100 George Street). Only at 45 Macquarie Street was there evidence of opiate-based cough medicine.

The church and medical reform

For centuries, churches were prominent advocates for health and wellness. The orthodox medical community began to threaten this role during the 19th century. This struggle is best portrayed in George Eliot's 1871 novel *Middlemarch, a study of provincial life* (set in the 1830s), a metaphorical contrast between the church and orthodox medicine in two characters: Casaubon, the ageing dusty cleric and Lydgate, the young doctor. In old age, Casaubon realises he is caught between his traditional theological beliefs and modern medicine. In contrast, young Lydgate embraces the dawning of positive science. This contrast is a metaphor for the movement to disconnect the church from a dominant position in medicine by the new positivism of science in medicine.[39]

In response to this threat, churches adapted in many ways, including establishing hospitals for orthodox medicine in which they tended to the physical and spiritual needs of the patients. The Parramatta Benevolent Society was formed in 1838 by Parramatta's clergy, Reverend Thomas Hassall and Reverend Mr Forrest, supported by Parramatta's philanthropists and other members of the clergy.[40] In 1848, when the society took over the operation of the Parramatta Hospital, it set aside the upper floor for the relief of female paupers.[41]

Churches also adopted a proactive approach to good health by promoting outdoor activities such as sporting events and social outings to pleasure grounds. The organisation of sport leagues has had a sustained impact on how Anglo-Christians view the relationship between sport, physical health (fitness) and religion.[42] Church social outings were a form of urban escapism that allowed city residents to travel outside the cities to experience a clean natural environment, if only for the day, to improve their overall wellness. Parramatta residents were fortunate to have the People's Park (later Parramatta Park), the domain around Government House that was gazetted in 1858. When the railway arrived at Parramatta in 1860, ready access to the coast expanded the range of church outings.

The two faces of Australian social class structure

In colonial New South Wales, social-class structure was an evolving precept prompted by its fragmented cultural origins, historical events, and shifting political and economic paradigms. Understanding how people functioned within this social structure has been instrumental in determining their compliance with Victorian values as they related to respectability and health. As a result of this study, it became apparent that there were two sides to their compliance – public and private – and based on levels of compliance, there was evidence of discrimination between the classes.

The public face of respectability

If respectability is the overarching goal of social reforms, then cleanliness is the thread that connects all aspects of Victorian values. Acceptable social etiquette and interaction in the public arena are important displays of

---

34 Grehan 2009, 55.
35 Potter 2017, 124.
36 Towler and Bramall 1986, 158.
37 Salt 1984, 121.
38 Cavender 2003, 107–11.

39 Chase 1991, 5.
40 *The Colonist* 21 February 1838, 2.
41 McClymont 1999.
42 D.W. Brown 1987; Watson, Weir and Friend 2005.

respectability, and "The individual necessarily provides a reading of himself when he is in the presence of others".[43]

Public alcohol consumption patterns represented social behaviours used to assess a person's respectability. These patterns are demonstrated in the archaeological record through a comparative analysis of alcohol and aerated water bottles from public houses located in Parramatta and other regional communities. The study results described above indicate that, by the late 19th century, Parramatta residents exhibited increased temperance in their public alcohol consumption and were more inclined to drink a non-alcoholic beverage, a pattern identified in other regional public house artefact collections. Eliminating negative behaviour patterns associated with public drunkenness was one reason for promoting temperance. Furthermore, many religious-based temperance movements promoted abstinence as a measure to achieve a clean body (internally), enabling a person to have a purity of soul.

Smoking in public was governed by several social constraints, most of which focused on women. Public smoking by females was socially unacceptable and smoking in the presence of a woman was discourteous. Pipe-smoking was so ingrained in colonial culture that many of the social conventions that discouraged smoking in other countries were not adhered to in colonial New South Wales.

Involvement in benevolent and religious institutions was a sign of respectability because these actions indicated virtue and a purity or cleanliness of the soul. Church attendance and participation in its various benevolent or social activities presented a public face of piety and respectability, yet they leave little evidence in the archaeological record. However, reported accounts in the newspapers and congregational newsletters often record social participation by case-study residents (as exemplified in Table 5.5 for site 4 and site 5 residents).

Proactive support for public health initiatives for a cleaner environment also contributed to a resident's respectability. In 19th-century Parramatta these initiatives included calls (reported by newspapers) for infrastructure reforms to better the community's health, temperance in public smoking, and health reforms.

The physical environment one lives in also expresses one's level of respectability. Where people lived was typically based on socio-economic position, which can be measured by characteristics such as income, occupation and education. The cleanliness of that environment was a factor in their choice of locations. Many areas of Parramatta had severe drainage problems that promoted mould and consequently threatened health. As this study shows, both working-class and some middle-class families lived in the lower-lying areas of town, while affluent middle-class gentry families lived on the well-drained alluvial terraces.

A closer examination of the patriarchs of the two middle-class gentry households provides information on how these properties were acquired. In 1799, Rowland Hassall (site 8) obtained a 14-year lease on a one-acre property on a well-drained alluvial slope. Reverend Hassall, an educated Methodist missionary, had financial resources, and when he moved to Parramatta, he brought with him materials to build a substantial stone dwelling, so he came with the three characteristic measures of middle-class status. At that time, all Parramatta properties were leased at the same 6 shillings per annum quit-rent, so the question remains: was preference given to affluent Rowland Hassall with the grant of this particular well-drained property? Unlike the land grant obtained by Hassall, in 1835 William Byrnes purchased his nearby well-drained property. Australian-born Williams Byrnes (site 6) was a successful Parramatta businessman with plans to build a steam-powered mill on the rivershoreline below his newly acquired property. With his wealth, Byrnes could afford to purchase several conjoined town lots in this preferred area.

The two semidetached houses (sites 4 and 5), erected by George Coates in the 1870s, were located on higher ground (above 12 metres) and had no drainage or severe mould issues. With their prominent preferred position, these dwellings were built on the eastern extent of D'Arcy Wentworth's subdivided estate. Wentworth was a highly regarded and influential government official in the late 18th century. In 1812 he received a 32-acre land grant in Parramatta on which he constructed Woodhouse, a fine manor house. These dwellings were tenanted by mostly middle-class professionals who could afford the rental costs in this desirable neighbourhood.

The private face of respectability

In contrast to the public face of respectability, Victorian values practised in the privacy of the home more accurately reflect actual attitudes to compliance with these values. Alcohol consumption and smoking are two practices that can be assessed in the archaeological record.

During the convict era (periods 1 and 2), temperance of alcohol consumption was seen as a step towards reforming behaviour within the convict population. Alcohol use and abuse was a measure of moral concern not only to those who opposed it. Those seeking to promote alcohol consumption had to work within the social and moral frameworks that moderate personal liberties and social tolerance. The etiquette of this period in the colony was to offer wine to guests at dinner, but if even one guest was known to hold temperance principles, then neither wine nor liquor should be brought to the table.[44]

There was a division in attitudes towards women's public and private alcohol consumptions as identified by Britain's 1877 Select Committee of the House of Lords

---

43 Beaudry, Cook and Mrozowski 1991, 277.

44 People's Publishing Company 1885, 128.

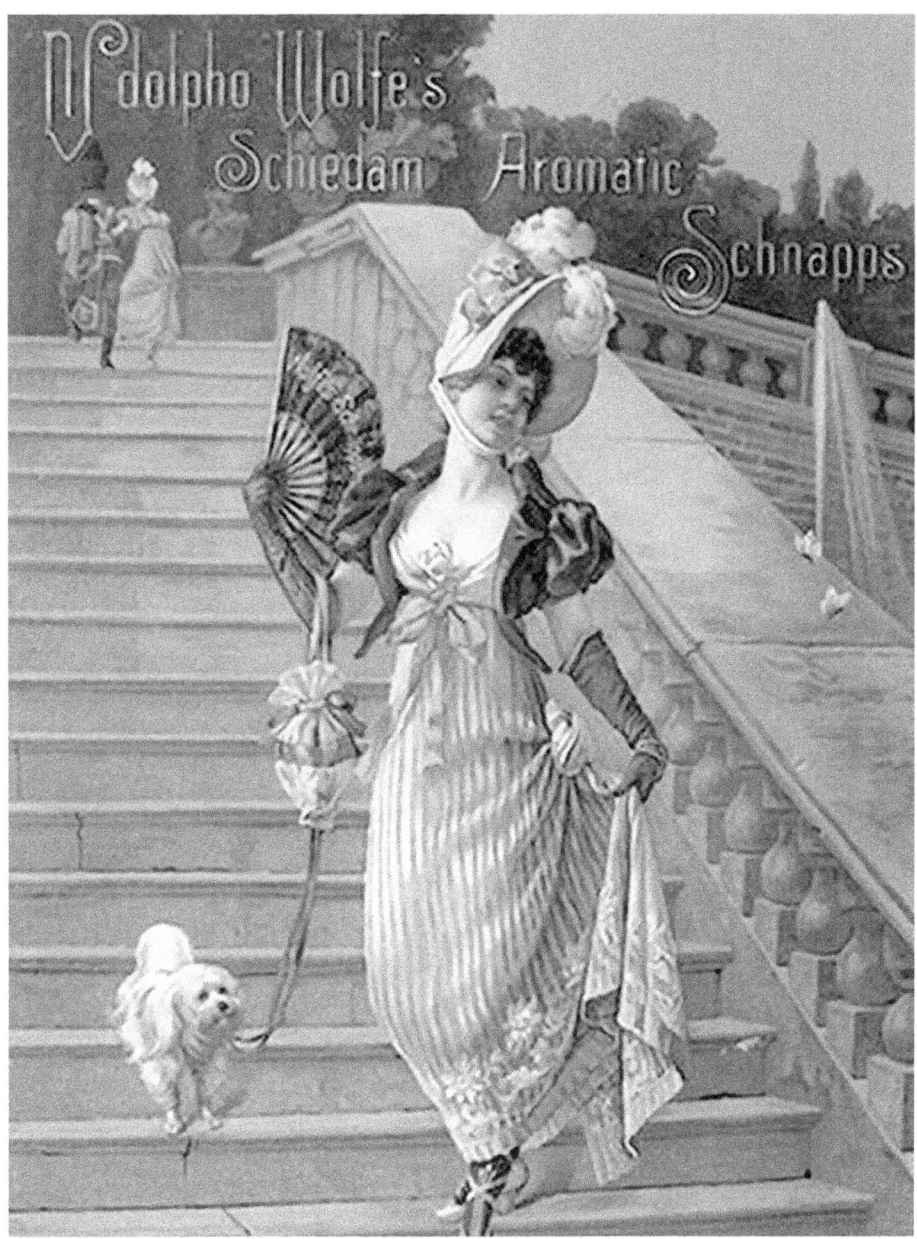

Figure 8.2 Late 19th century Udolpho Wolfe trade card (with recipes on reverse side).

on Intemperance. Public drinking was linked to vice and often crime, while in-home middle-class drinking was considered personal preference, much like food choices.[45] In many households, medicinal alcohol was a means of social compliance with temperance values, while still imbibing alcohol. Wine and schnapps were alcoholic beverages often used for medicinal purposes. Medicinal alcohol was often prescribed by doctors to women with female physiological and nervous complaints, and often with the husband's encouragement. More often than not wine was prescribed, but widely advertised medicinal schnapps was also imbibed. Schnapps advertising targeted the female market (Figure 8.2). Often women drank in solitude and secrecy.[46] The home was a woman's domain and where she spent the majority of her time. Substance abuse among women is exemplified within the home. There was a noticeable increase in the consumption of schnapps for half of the case-study assemblages that post-date 1860 (Table 7.11), which coincidently is the year Udolpho Wolfe launched his aggressive marketing campaign for medicinal schnapps throughout the colonies.

In-home alcohol consumption practices during the 19th century experienced changing patterns, but not necessarily decreases in consumption. The difference between public and private drinking patterns is an obvious example of this difference between public and private faces of

---

45 Hands 2018, 41.

46 Murdock 1998, 44–6.

Cleanliness is next to godliness

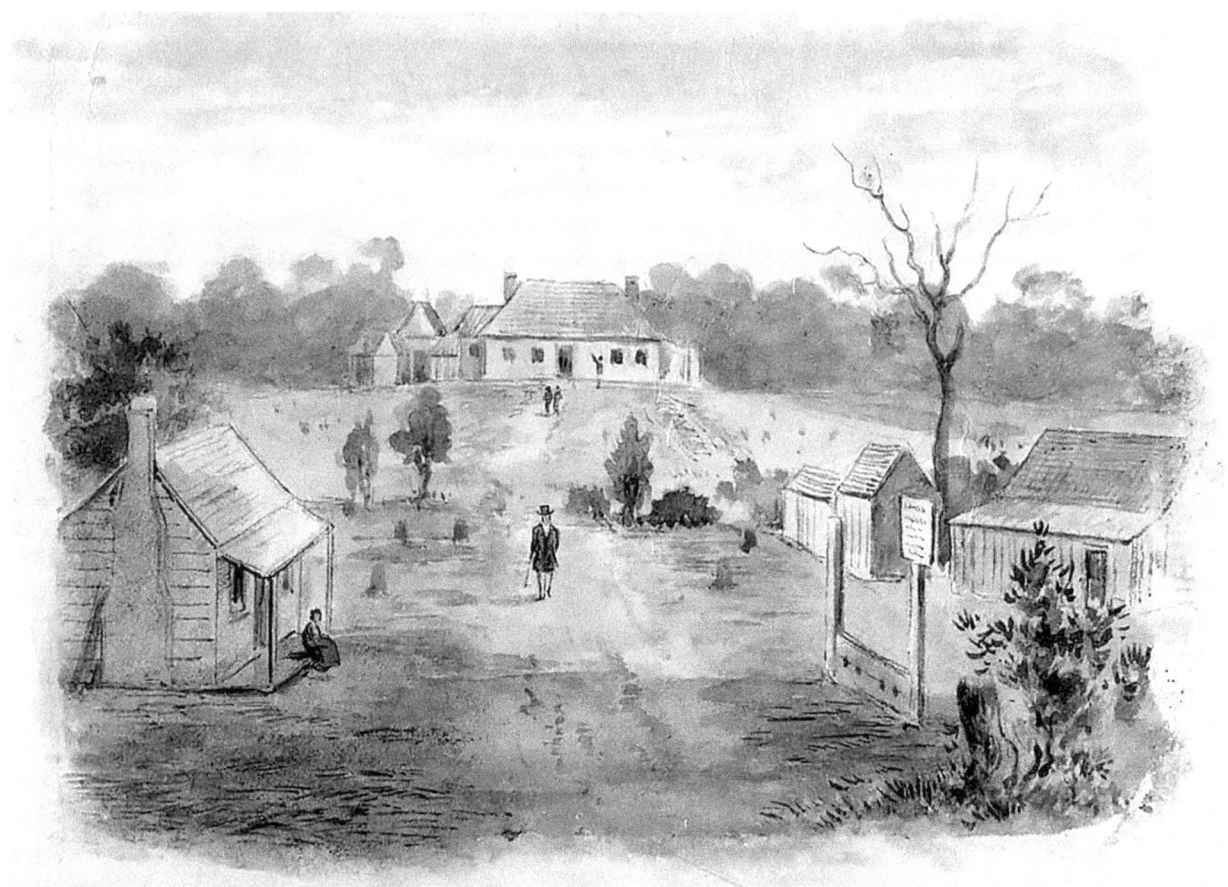

Figure 8.3 View of Parramatta looking towards the Governor's House (1798). Source: Dixson Galleries, State Library of New South Wales (DG SSV1A/11).

respectability. Until the 1860s, both public and private drink habits were 100 per cent alcohol. Between 1860 and 1890, the relative frequency of alcohol consumption in public houses dropped from 100 per cent to 34.5 per cent. For middle-class gentry homes (sites 6 and 8), the relative frequency of alcohol consumed during this time ranged from 88.9 to 94.9 per cent, but, in the one middle-class household in this timeframe, the relative frequency was 100 per cent. Alcohol consumption patterns differ for the two semidetached homes on Taylor Street (sites 4 and 5); one dropped only slightly to 83.6 per cent (1890–1920), while the other dropped to 45.5 per cent (1900–1935).

In-home smoking practices varied throughout the 19th century. During the late 18th century and early 19th century, the limited tobacco supply probably influenced the low relative frequencies of pipes in the earliest case-study assemblages (sites 6 and 7). The increased availability of locally-grown tobacco during the 1820s is reflected in the increased relative frequency of clay pipes in the 1823–1841 working-class assemblage of site 2. From the mid-19th century, the marked decline in tobacco consumption reflects temperance movements' increased influence over in-home smoking practices.

Discrimination towards the disrespectable

Discrimination is the prejudicial treatment of different categories of people based on set, preconceived criteria. Class distinctions are viewed in terms of personal qualities. Social class is just one of many manifestations of class structure. Previously, there was an inference that social conformity to Victorian values resulted from social pressures, but the archaeological record cannot determine if non-compliance with these standards led to discrimination. Signs of discrimination come from historical research and examination of the historical record.

When the first convicts arrived in New South Wales, the concept that everyone deserves a fair go was an ideology at least 50 years in the colony's future. During those first 50 years, discrimination towards emancipists and convicts was evident in all aspects of life in the colony. Governor Macquarie's (1810–1821) policy for equality of every emancipist was resisted and rejected by military and civilian officers, and free settlers.[47] The social discrimination by the middle class of successful female emancipists, such as businesswoman Mary Reibey and the wealthy daughter of emancipists, Sarah Wentworth, typifies the general attitudes of the free

---

47 Karskens 2010, 225.

8 Colonial Parramatta: a medical anthropological approach to health and class

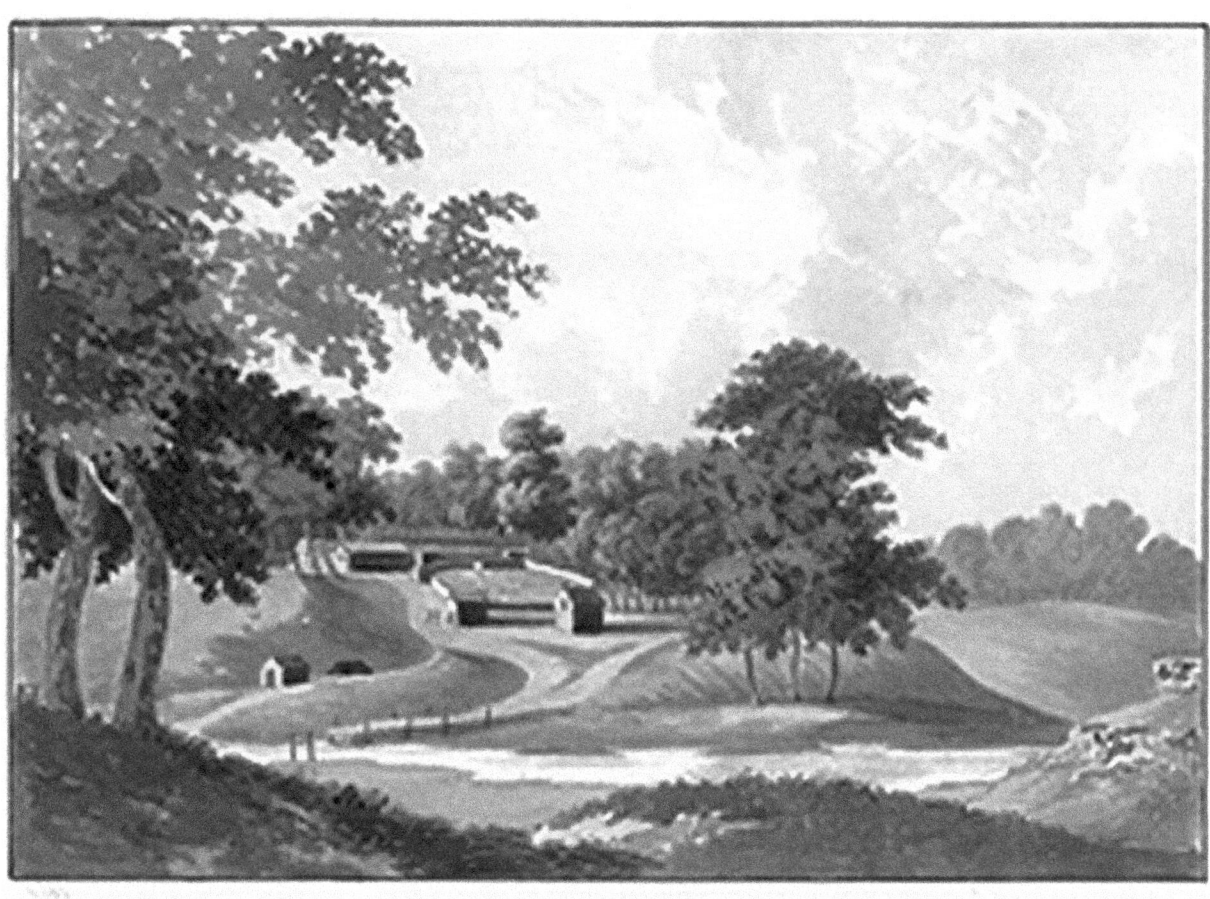

Figure 8.4 View of the redoubt at Rose Hill, drawn by E. Dayes from a sketch by J. Hunter. Source: National Library of Australia (Rex Nan Kivell Collection NK2766/B).

segment of the population. For convicts, the situation was much worse. While the 1828 *Masters and Servants Act* provided for equality in the workplace, most convicts were unacceptable on a social level to other classes.

Female convicts were generally regarded as disreputable "whores" because they failed to exhibit the mannerisms associated with middle-class propriety. Furthermore, they were seen as prostitutes for living in de facto relationships, relationships that afforded female convicts protection against sexual assaults. In order to wed, a convict must have first received government permission and then pay the often-prohibitive cost for a marriage licence, so many therefore chose a de facto relationship.

There was discrimination within the ranks of convictism. For example, while the class system imposed at the Parramatta Female Factory was initially based on the nature of the crime the inmate was serving a sentence for, lesser offenders could have their privileges revoked if they were disrespectful or dirty. A hierarchy also existed among the male convict community. Gentlemen convicts were those with skill sets or British-based social status that afforded them assignments within the government's operating structure and ultimately earned them pardons.

Where they lived

Parramatta's original town layout situated the governor's home on the high ground at the western end of High Street (later George Street) overlooking convict huts located along the low-lying section of the street, with the redoubt at the eastern end of High Street on the well-drained alluvial slope above the Parramatta River (Figures 8.3 and 8.4). It is probably not a coincidence that the two middle-class gentry residents' homes in the case study were located on this well-drained alluvial slope. As noted, in 1799, highly respected Reverend Rowland Hassall acquired a a well-drained one-acre property. It could be assumed that Hassall's status and plans to build a substantial two-story brick home in Parramatta afforded him this privileged location. By the time William Byrnes purchased the lots at the corner of George and Charles streets in 1838, he and his brother James operated a successful steam ferry transport service between Parramatta and Sydney and they soon erected a flour mill on the riverbank next to the landing-place wharf. The proximity of Byrnes' house lots to his business interests was probably intentional, and given his financial stability, he could afford the cost of this prime location.

Where they obtained health care

Discrimination is evident in Parramatta's healthcare system during the convict era. The medical services available to convicts and free settlers included access to hospital facilities. Yet even non-convict paupers refused to be admitted to the Parramatta Hospital because it meant association with the convict patients. Shortly after transportation to New South Wales ended in 1840, Parramatta Hospital was transferred from government to local committee management in 1848. The subsequent segregated floors for convicts and free settlers alleviated the problem of common wards for convicts and non-convicts. Nevertheless, this change still represented discrimination because while the convicts were still treated by government medical staff, free settlers were administered by a benevolent society attending to the health of mostly female paupers. The Parramatta Female Factory had a lying-in hospital staffed with certified surgeons and midwives, yet most free female settlers in Parramatta did not use these facilities. The only free women recorded as using the Female Factory lying-in hospital services were Mary Morrissy and Rosanne Kelly.[48] Both women were ex-convicts who had obtained their tickets of freedom, and both of them lost a child during delivery, which may imply that besides convict mothers, only emancipated working-class women experiencing difficulty in delivery used the factory's hospital facilities. Still, in the late 19th century, many wives of middle-class gentry settlers, such as Mrs Marsden and Mrs Macarthur, chose to travel to Sydney to be tended in private lying-in facilities. Other middle-class gentry wives, such as Mrs Hassell (site 8), had their children at home, while others like Mrs Pringle (site 6) and Mrs Oakes delivered their babies at the Parramatta Hospital.

When the government ceased providing medical care for all in the 1840s, private medical care was expensive due partly to the limited number of medical practitioners. In 1830, Parramatta had one physician in private practice, William Sherwin, to tend to nearly 3,000 free settlers. While the number of private-practice surgeries increased to 10 by 1850 (to service a population of over 4,000), the fees were still prohibitive to the working class and poor.

The New South Wales colony was always proactive in charitable and governmental support for the infirm, aged, destitute and insane. In Parramatta alone, there was the Government Benevolent Asylum (George Street), the Hospital for the Insane (Factory Street) and the Infirm and Destitute Asylum (Macquarie Street). Yet, for nearly 50 years (1840–1890), Parramatta's working class found themselves situated between the middle class who could afford the expense of private medical care and the very needy who were looked after by benevolent societies and government agencies. Due to their financial situation, the working class and poor had limited access to medical treatment. The first affordable medical care for the working class in Parramatta came with the 1890 formation of the Parramatta and District United Friendly Societies' Dispensary and Medical Institute. The need for these services was so great that when the 1902 influenza epidemic broke out in Parramatta, the demand for prescriptions depleted the dispensary's funds.[49] Other voluntary health insurance schemes developed during the early 20th century, but not until the government introduced universal Medicare in 1975 did the working class truly have access to affordable health care.

---

48 Reese 1991, 119, 157.

49 *Sydney Morning Herald* 25 January 1902, 12.

CONCLUDING REMARKS

Parramatta's emerging middle class during the early colonial period in New South Wales grew to be the prevailing social class by the end of the 19th century. Its socio-economic position in society gave the middle class power to impose its values on its peers and the mostly working-class population. Victorian values for social reform emulate attributes of moral and social respectability that are, in fact, guidelines for improved health practices. Archaeological and historical scholarship generally interprets respectability as a marker of the socio-economic status of the middle class, however, good health practices were the underlying principle for these values. Furthermore, the thread of cleanliness connects the values of sobriety, piety, work ethic and chastity, for a clean lifestyle is ultimately viewed as a respectable lifestyle.

At the beginning of this research, the question was asked: "What evidence of consistent agency is apparent for the health care of Parramatta's residents?" The use of an interdisciplinary approach facilitated a broad-spectrum interpretation that Parramatta residents were more than passive adherents to the social conventions set out as Victorian values. The argument that these values have a proactive effect on personal health is validated through sociological studies, historical records and medical reforms. This holistic research methodology presents a more comprehensive view of their cultural impact on health. What remains to be determined is whether individual adherence to these values was purposeful in terms of measures for improved health or compliance measures to obtain the desired respectability status. The archaeological record provides complementary insight into this line of inquiry.

Using a city-wide perspective demonstrates the utility of systematic synthesis of archaeological data. Including multiple sites representing Parramatta's four 19th-century time periods with representation from the three major social classes facilitates a broader community perspective for data interpretation. One of the outcomes is identifying dichotomous alcohol consumption patterns that developed for public drinking habits and in-home consumption of alcohol. Drinking was as much a social ritual as a coping mechanism to reduce anxiety in the New South Wales colonial environment. When they came in the mid-19th century, changes to these drinking habits were influenced by temperance movements. In Parramatta, the dramatic drop in drinking in public houses indicates that people adopted a public face of alcohol temperance. At the same time, their in-home drinking practices lessened only slightly, with some residents even disguising their drinking by dosing with medicinal alcohol. By the early 20th century, statistics for in-home alcohol consumption were substantially lower than those of late 19th-century households, demonstrating a significant shift towards temperance and sobriety in drinking habits.

Some aspects of artefact analysis produced limited results for my research questions. Tobacco pipes were used to assess levels of social compliance for smoking habits. However, historical research indicates that tobacco sourcing and supply during early colonial times (c. 1790–1830) affected tobacco use more than the social pressures for temperance. Furthermore, analysis of smoking pipes was possible for collections that post-date the stabilisation of the tobacco supply. For the remainder of the long 19th century, temperance movements' social pressures in all social classes influenced the decline in smoking, culminating with a cessation of pipe-smoking in late 19th to early 20th-century households.

Not all aspects of artefact analysis produced conclusive results. Many patent medicines represented in the study had multiple applications and could not be linked with treatment for a specific ailment. Furthermore, the research strategy used for this book was designed to demonstrate in-home medical practices, but the sample was based mostly on post-1860s embossed-labelled bottles. It, therefore, did not adequately address self-medication practices for the early 19th-century case-study households. It failed to distinguish any significant differences in approach to self-medication between social classes, and it failed to determine an increase or decrease in orthodox medicine use throughout the 19th century.

Evidence for environmental reforms for improved health in the community is documented in the historical record and supported in the archaeological record. In Parramatta, infrastructure reforms for clean water supply were initiated on both a local and colonial basis in response to repeated calls in the media from middle-class citizens. Dams that represented early efforts are still intact and remnants of the 1900s water and sewerage scheme are evidenced during most archaeological excavations in the town. Public health reforms for the control and eradication of contagious diseases were colonial initiatives. The first of these initiatives, smallpox inoculations, originated in Parramatta. Implementing widespread inoculation in New South Wales was the subject of debate in the media on both a colonial and local basis.

A theme that emerged throughout this research is discrimination against convicts, emancipists and the working class that affected their health. By virtue of their criminal background, convicts and emancipists were subject to widespread social discrimination from the working and middle classes despite their economic success or their efforts to conform to social conventions of respectability. Discrimination, based on socio-economic factors, influenced where the working class lived. Parramatta's working class lived in the predominantly low-lying, damp-ridden areas of the town, while at the other end of the social spectrum the middle-class gentry lived in the town's well-drained areas. Furthermore, the lower economic status of the working class detrimentally affected their ability to obtain affordable health care, and this lack of availability influenced their preference for self-medication with patent medicines.

This research is the first scholarly work to present the archaeology and history of Victorian social conventions as something more than respectability manifested as socio-economic status, manners and etiquette. These values – sobriety, piety, work ethic and chastity – are tied together by cleanliness, and so are standards that influenced attitudes towards health for all classes of colonial society. This novel interpretation centred on cleanliness and health offers an additional consideration in future archaeological studies that address Victorian values.

APPENDIX: SITES IN THE CASE STUDY

Sites considered for the case study were assessed for their ability to meet the parameters outlined in Chapter 3. The eight sites selected for inclusion each contained a sealed and dated feature deposit that corresponded to a documented occupant of that site (Table A.1). Selection also represented the different time periods in Parramatta's past (see Table 2.1). Furthermore, consideration was given to geographic location within the town to provide a representation of differing approaches to addressing drainage issues (Figure A.1).

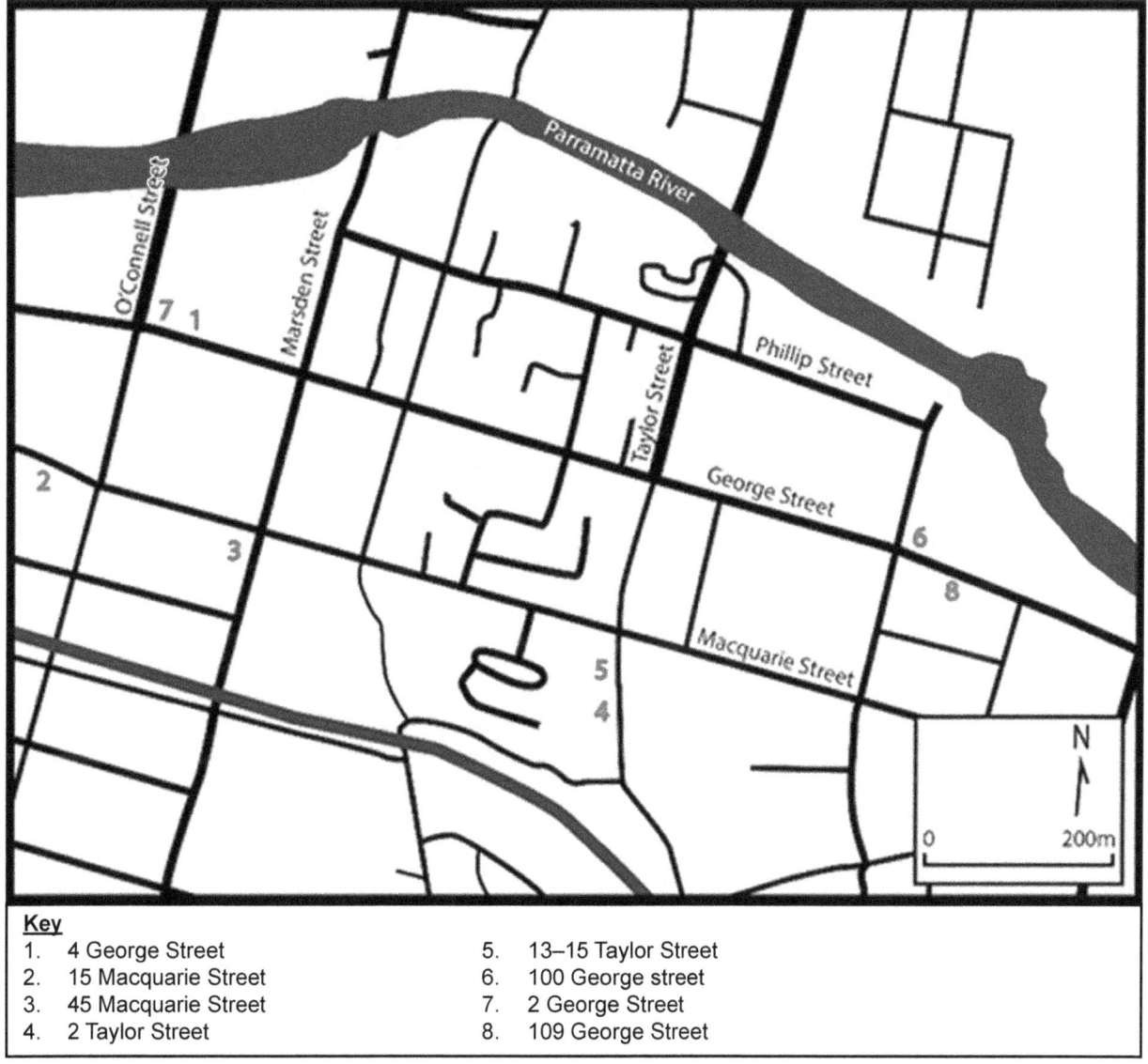

Key
1. 4 George Street
2. 15 Macquarie Street
3. 45 Macquarie Street
4. 2 Taylor Street
5. 13–15 Taylor Street
6. 100 George street
7. 2 George Street
8. 109 George Street

Figure A.1 Plan of Parramatta showing the locations of sites in the case study.

Cleanliness is next to godliness

Table A.1 Summary information for features at case-study sites.

Site No.	Address	Feature type	Owner/Resident	Date range	Archaeological Project
1	4 George St	Cesspit 6024	James McRoberts	1820–1860	Parramatta Justice Precinct
1	4 George St	Cesspit 6039	James McRoberts	1830–1870	Parramatta Justice Precinct
2	15 Macquarie St	Dam/pond	John Noble	1823–1841	15 Macquarie Street
3	45 Macquarie St	Well	Walker/Sweeney	1860–1880	Marsden & Macquarie Sts
4	2 Taylor St	North cistern	Henry Byrnes	1890s–1920	1 Smith Street
5	13–15 Taylor St	Cistern	Tenanted	1890–1930	143–169 Macquarie St
6	100 George St	Pit	Thomas Halfpenny	1790–1830	George & Charles Sts
6	100 George St	Well 2417	Byrnes Family	1830–1920	George & Charles Sts
6	100 George St	Cesspit 2206	Byrnes Family	1860–1940	George & Charles Sts
6	100 George St	Cesspit 2369	Byrnes Family	1840–1890	George & Charles Sts
6	100 George St	Cesspit 2370	Byrnes Family	1840–1890	George & Charles Sts
7	2 George St	Cellar	Samuel Larkin	1810–1840s	Parramatta Children's Court
8	109 George St	Well	Hassell Family	1810–1840s	109–113 George Street
8	109 George St	Rubbish pit	Hassell Family	1820–1880	109–113 George Street

Site 1: 4 George Street

Historically, 4 George Street was designated as Lot 99 George Street. It is bound to the south by George Street, to the east by Lot 98 and to the west by Lot 102 with a creek line crossing the property's north-west corner. The site's first occupation was a timber hut that was built during the 1790s and occupied by convicts until 1806, when the Crown leased it to free settlers. James Harrex received a land grant for Lot 99 in approximately 1806. Harrex lived at the property until his death in 1825; records indicate it was tenanted from 1831 to 1837. In 1837 a stone house was constructed fronting George Street. The following year, Harrex's daughter Hannah Sarah married James McRoberts. When the estate was portioned in 1847 "Sarah" McRoberts acquired the property. The McRoberts family occupied this property from 1855 to 1862. James Garvey lived there from 1862 to 1873; it was occupied finally by Isaac and Bridget King from 1873 to 1916.[1]

The deposit selected for this site is from a cesspit (Context 6024), located at the rear of the lot (Figure A.2), that contained 2,561 artefacts representing 465 minimum item count (MIC). The cesspit deposit was excavated in four arbitrary spits (levels) in order to identify any temporal distinctions. However, the mixed temporal nature of artefacts from these spits (top to bottom) within the cesspit indicates there was no discernible temporal difference in stratigraphy. Approximately 71 per cent of artefacts provided temporal data that was used to establish a 1780s–1860s date range for the deposit. Analysis results indicate the deposit was sealed by the 1870s. Approximately 18 per cent of the artefacts date specifically to the convict and emancipated convict era of site development and the remainder date from the McRoberts occupation of the site. It is most likely the cesspit fill is a result of yard or site clean-up activities between the occupation of the site by McRoberts and Garvey.

---

1   Miskella 2005, 7; Casey & Lowe 2005b, 3.

Appendix: sites in the case study

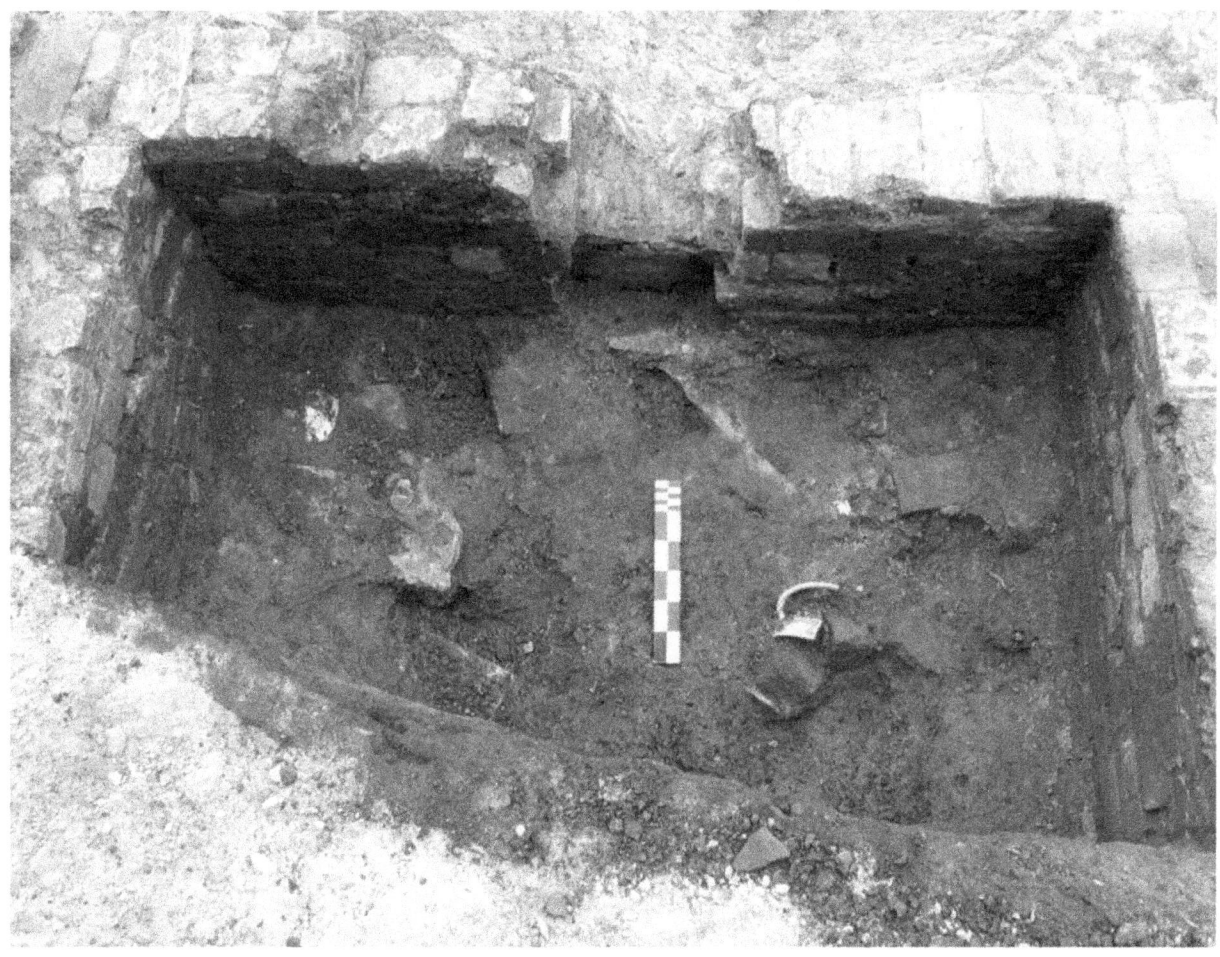

Figure A.2 Cesspit at 4 George Street (site 1) that is used in the case study. Source: Miskella 2005, 17.

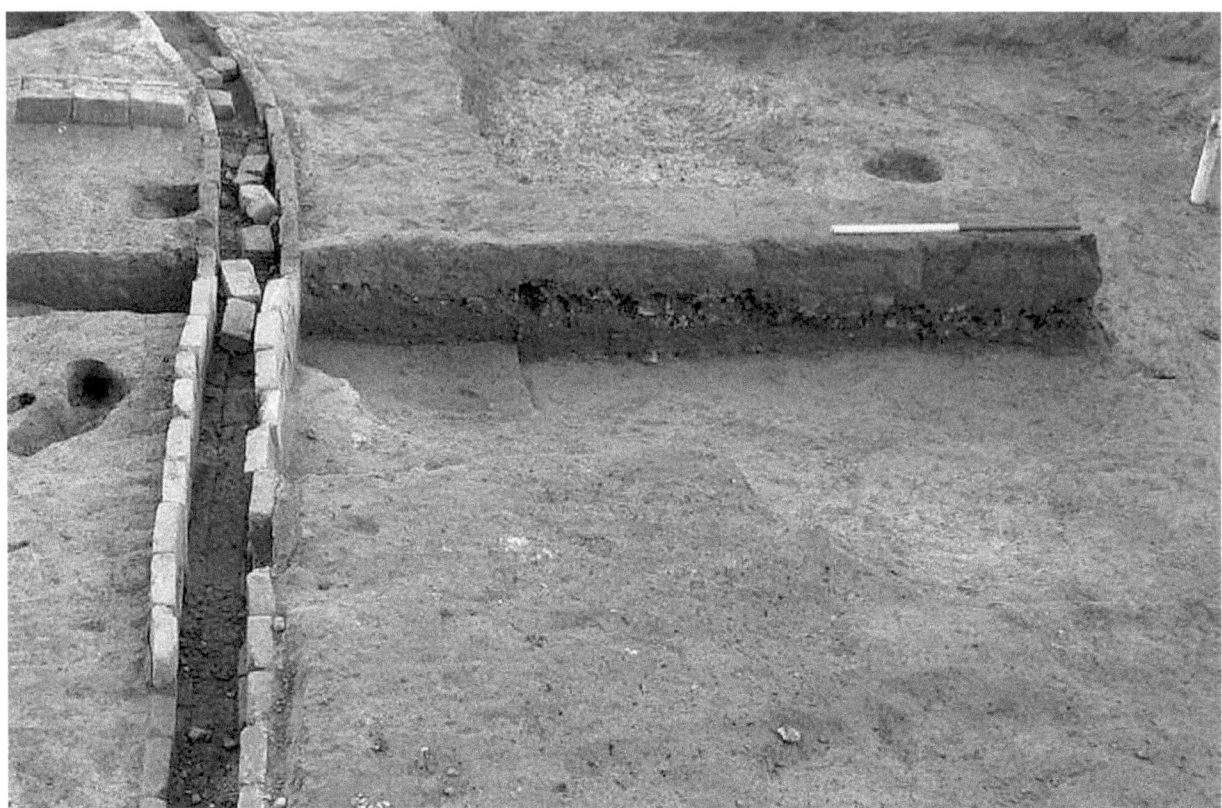

Figure A.3 Early drain and partially excavated pond at 15 Macquarie Street (site 2). Source Casey & Lowe 2012, 51.

Site 2: 15 Macquarie Street

As early as 1793 the property at 15 Macquarie (Lot 7, Section 11) was cleared and used for agricultural purposes, as evidenced in the archaeological record by hoe marks and rudimentary drainage channels. By 1804, when formal allotments were designated, a timber structure occupied the property, set back on the lot behind a natural pond. The pond was modified, and a dam and drains were constructed to combat the drainage problems present on this low-lying property (Figure A.3). This structure was still standing when ticket-of-leave holder John Noble formally leased the property in 1823, although he may have lived there as early as his first convict assignment in 1814. There was archaeological evidence that Noble deliberately backfilled the pond, with rubbish and soil, during his occupancy of the property (1823–1841).[2] A total of 4,973 artefacts representing 2,511 MIC were recovered from this feature. The backfill was conducted in a series of distinct episodes, which artefact analysis results could determine had an only slight temporal variation; early deposits were assigned with an overall 1800–1835 date range and an 1823–1860 date range was assigned to the uppermost historic topsoil deposit.

---

2   Casey & Lowe 2012, 107.

Appendix: sites in the case study

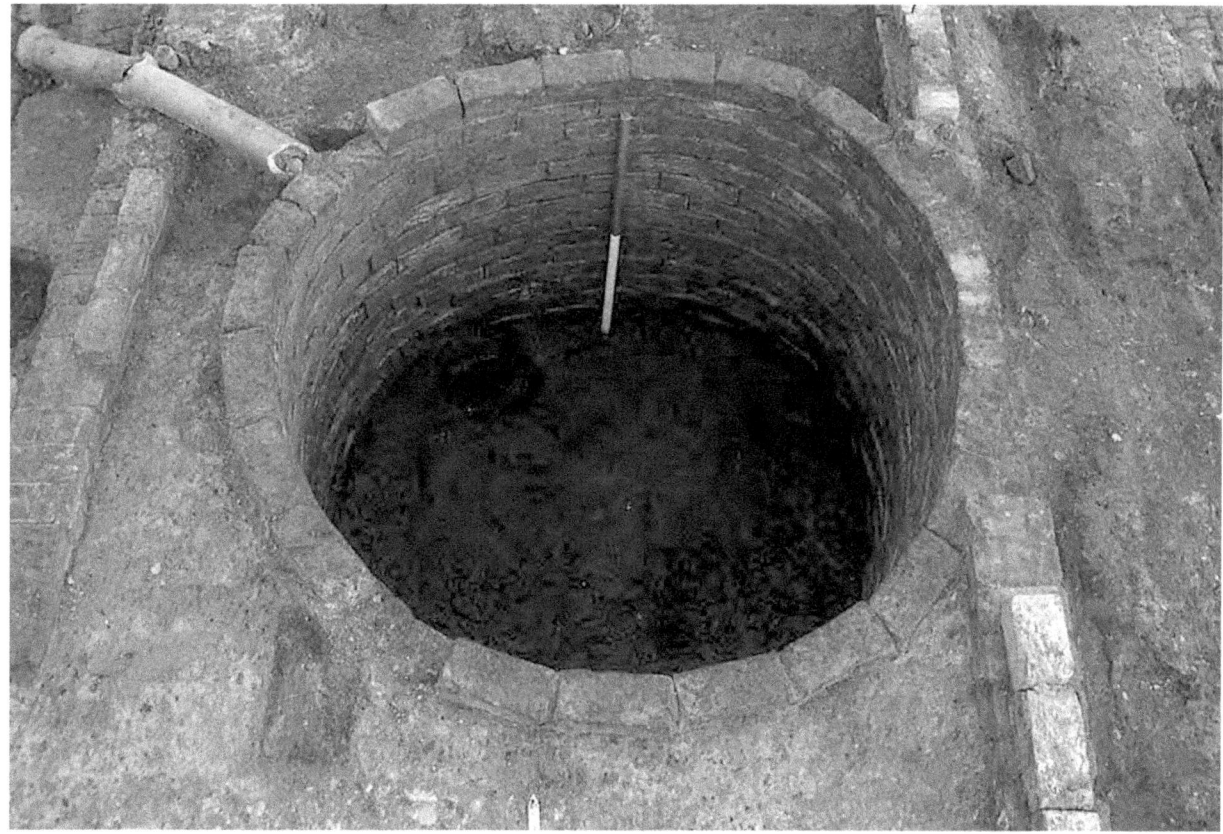

Figure A.4 Well at the rear of 45 Macquarie Street (site 3) that is used in the case-study. Source: Higginbotham 2007.

Site 3: 45 Macquarie Street

The archaeological excavations at 45 Macquarie Street delineated remains of a brick house built in the 1830s. The house was located on an alluvial floodplain near the western limits of the town. At the rear of this property (Allotment 16) was a sandstock brick-lined well (Context 649) (Figure A.4). (The bricks used to construct the well are identical to those used in the construction of the house.) The 2007 archaeological investigation indicated that the well was contemporaneous with the house, and therefore it was in service from the 1830s.[3] According to town plans from the late 1870s or early 1880s, the well was covered by an outbuilding. The well shaft, which measured 1.7 metres in diameter, was excavated to a depth of 1.2 metres, at which point excavation was discontinued (Figure A.4). A total of 3,227 artefacts representing 881 MIC were recovered from this feature. Based on temporal data for artefacts recovered from well deposits, the original archaeological interpretation suggested that the well continued in service until the 1890s. Re-evaluation indicates it was abandoned in the 1870s when the outbuilding overlaid it. It was subsequently used for rubbish disposal from that time until the late 1890s.

---

3   Higginbotham 2007, 18.

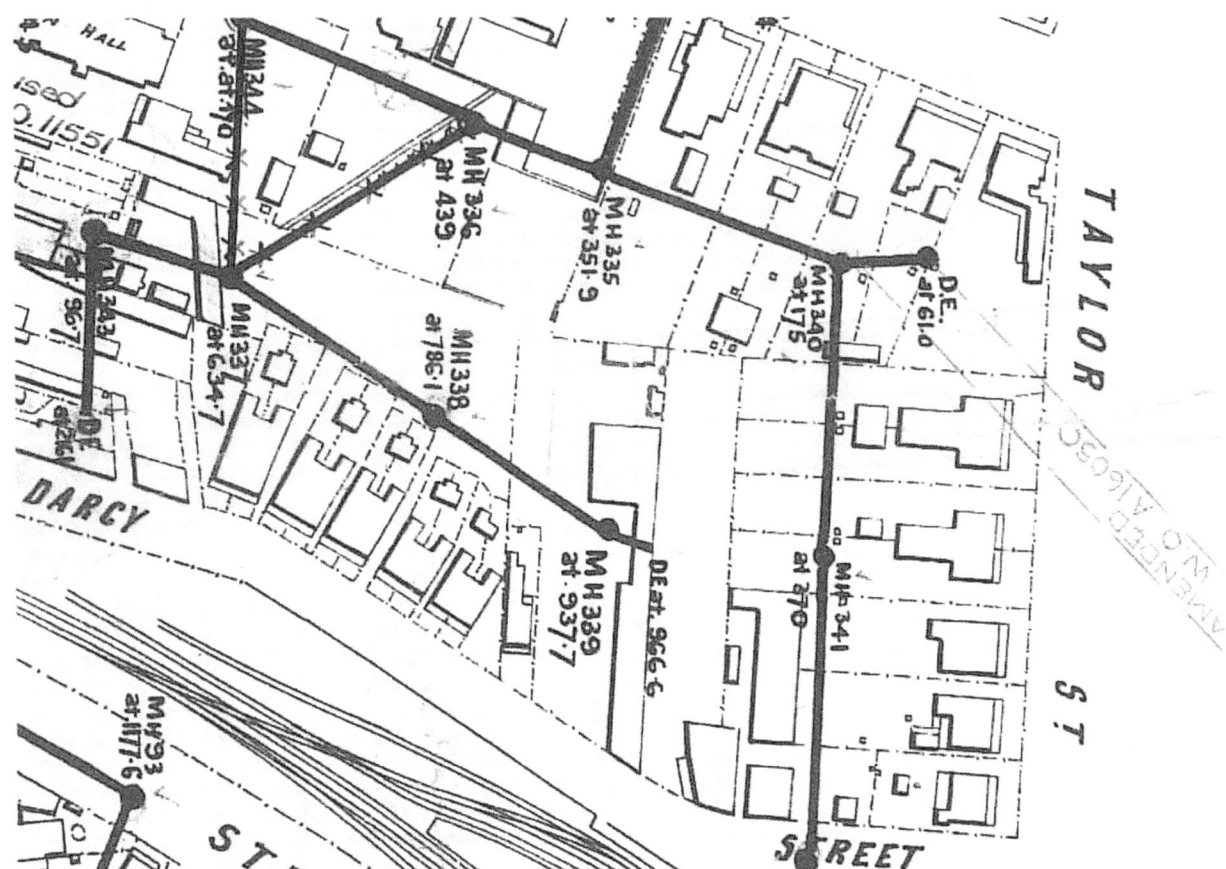

Figure A.5 A 1907 Sydney Water map showing semidetached dwellings on the west side of Taylor Street (sites 4–5).

Sites 4–5: Wentworth Estate, 2 and 13–15 Taylor Street

The "Wentworth Estate" was a large land grant in south Parramatta and the site of D'Arcy Wentworth's Woodhouse home. After the mid-1870s subdivision of the property (also called the Wentworth Estate), builder and property developer George Coates constructed five structures consisting of three detached houses and two semidetached dwellings, on the western side of the new southern extension to Taylor Street (now Smith Street) between Macquarie and D'Arcy streets.

Archaeological investigations have been conducted at several residences within the Wentworth Estate, including a detached residence at 2 Taylor Street and a semidetached residence at 13–15 Taylor Street[4] (Figure A.5). Two beehive cisterns located at the rear of these properties were selected for inclusion in this case study (Figures A.6 and A.7). The cisterns were abandoned when the municipal water supply was installed, which was first recorded on the Sydney Water Department map in 1907.[5] The cistern at 2 Taylor Street was excavated entirely to a depth of 2.95 metres. A total of 395 artefacts representing 307 MIC were recovered from this feature. The cistern at the rear of 13–15 Taylor Street contained a total of 358 artefacts representing 268 MIC. Both were filled with secondary deposition characterised as a site clean-up – possibly between occupancies.

---

4 Casey & Lowe 2005.
5 Aird 1961, 161–3.

Appendix: sites in the case study

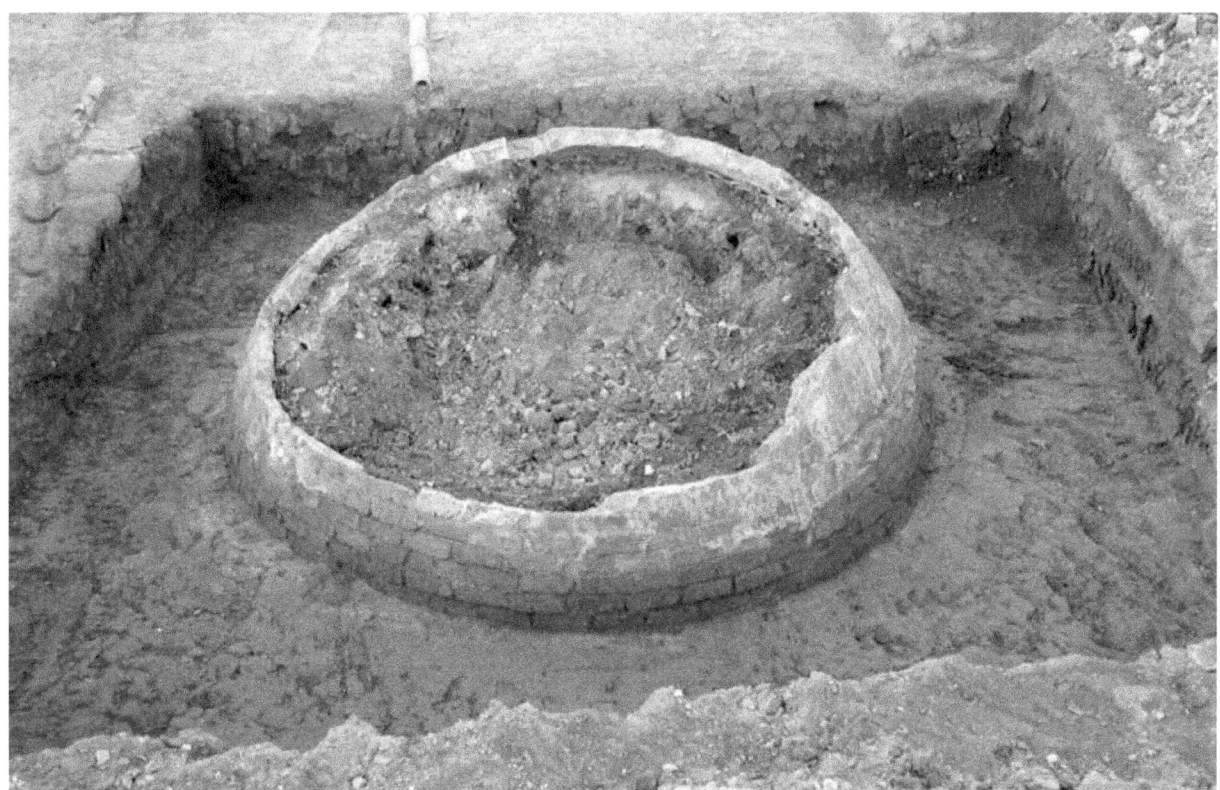

Figure A.6 Northern cistern at the rear of 2 Taylor Street (site 4). Source: Casey & Lowe 2005a, 24.

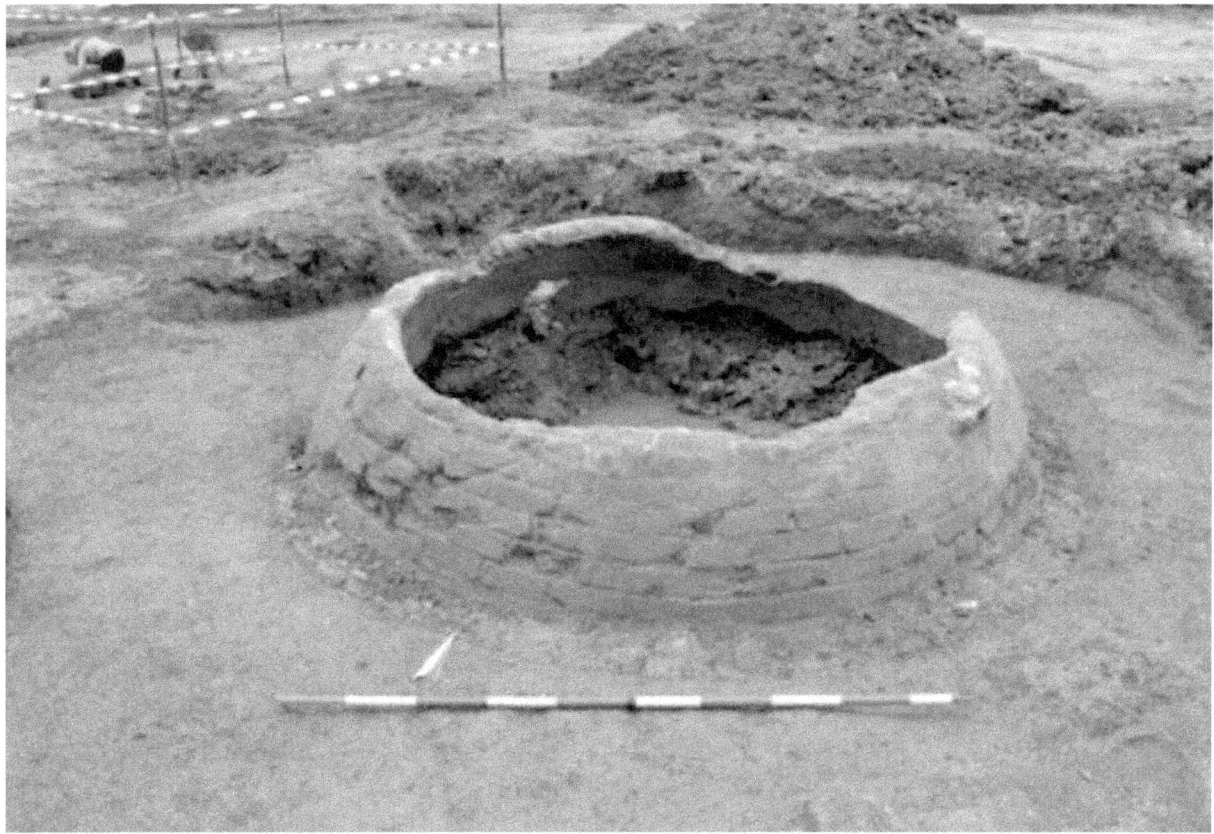

Figure A.7 Cistern at the rear of 15 Taylor Street (site 5). Source: GML Heritage 2015, 51.

Table A.2. Summary information for features from 100 George Street used in the case study.

Feature type	Allotment	Context #	Date range	Quantity	MIC
Rubbish pit	14	1691	1790–1830	228	98
Cesspit	70	2369	1840–90	2587	1137
Cesspit	70	2206	1860–1930	1077	513
Cesspit	70	2370	1840–90	1016	271
Well	69	2417	1830–90	2935	1533

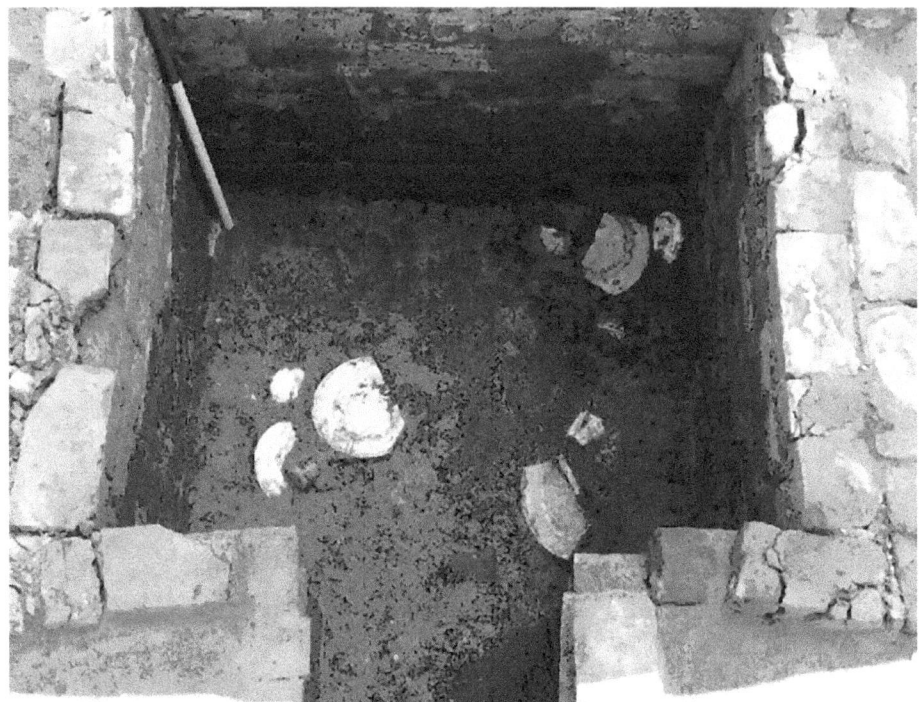

Figure A.8 Cesspit (site 6). Allotment 70, 100 George Street, used in the case study. Source: Miskella 2003, 9.

Site 6: 100 George Street

In 1823, the property was designated as seven allotments (13, 14, 16, 18, 69, 70 and 72) with all lots situated on a sandy alluvial terrace overlooking the Parramatta River. The lots were identified as 100–102 George Street in the late 19th century and were renumbered to 180–180a during the 20th century. Convict huts were built on all lots by 1804, but the occupants were not recorded. When the first documented occupant, Thomas Halfpenny, obtained a 14-year lease in 1804, the property was considered as a whole and yet was recorded as divided into allotments. An ex-marine and free settler, Halfpenny split his time between his rented 7-acre farm on the Hawkesbury and Parramatta. He died in 1810, and the auction notice for the property listed a 5-bedroom shingled and weatherboard house. Little is known of Walter Lawry, who owned the property from 1823 until William Byrnes purchased the property in 1838 and constructed a large stone manor house.[6] The Byrnes sisters, Emmeline and Marian, lived most of their lives in the Georgian manor that their father William built on the north-east corner of George and Charles streets in the 1830s.

Five features from this site are used in the case study (Table A.2). They represent different phases of the site's occupation. An early 19th-century rubbish pit (Context 1691), located near the north-east boundary of Lot 14, is one of a series of pits associated with a dwelling located north of Lot 14. Temporal data for artefacts from this rubbish pit are consistent with Halfpenny's occupation of the site. Two mid-19th-century brick-lined cesspits (2369 and 2370) were located on the south half of Lot 70, an allotment that, from the time of the Byrnes occupation, was an ornamental garden in the front and a kitchen garden in the rear. One late 19th-century cesspit (2206) was also located on the south half of Lot 70 (Figures A.8 and A.9). An early-to late-19th-century well was located on Lot 69 (Figure A.10).

---

6 Kass 2002, 5.

Appendix: sites in the case study

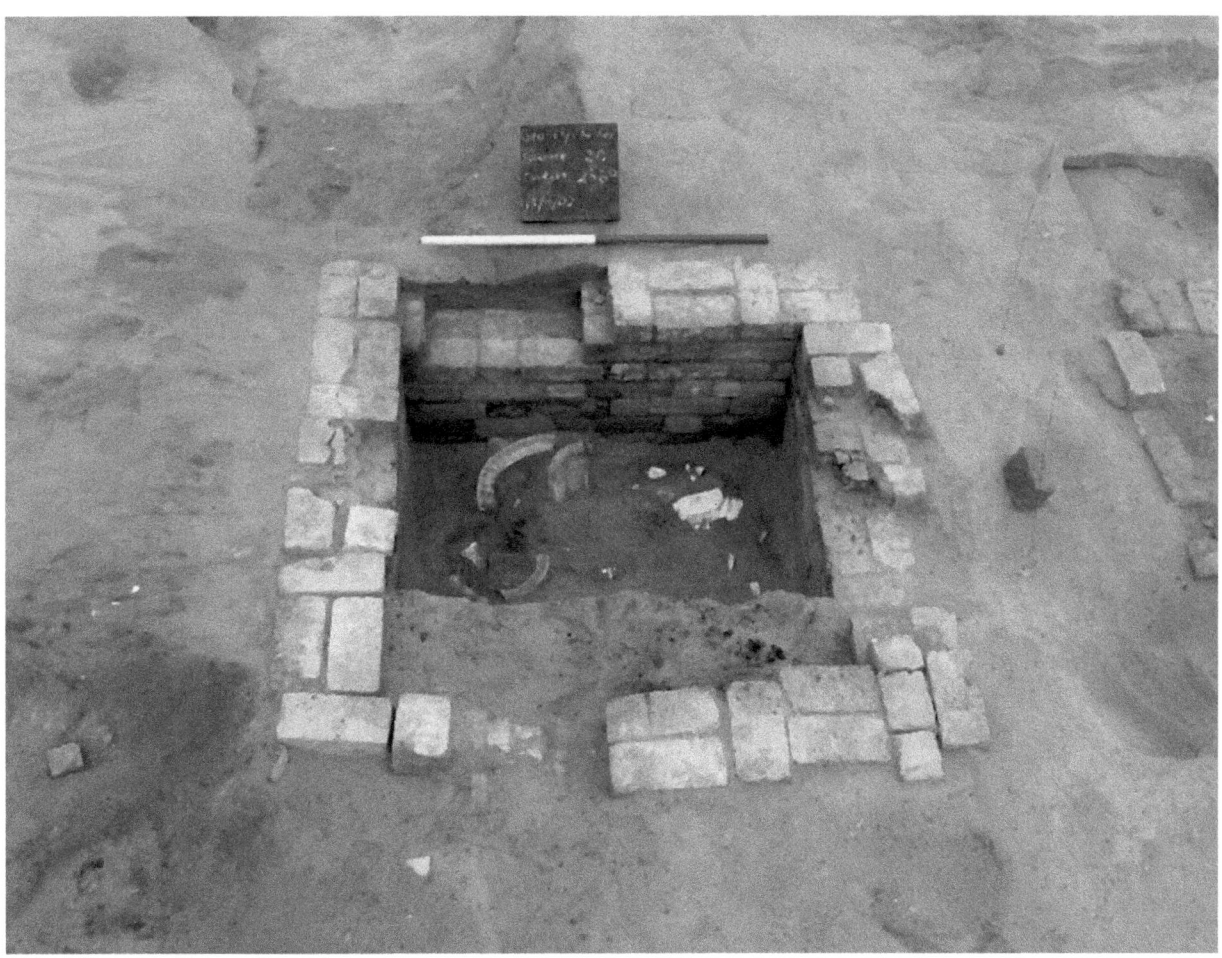

Figure A.9 Cesspit (site 6). Allotment 70, 100 George Street, used in the case study. Source: Miskella 2003, 9.

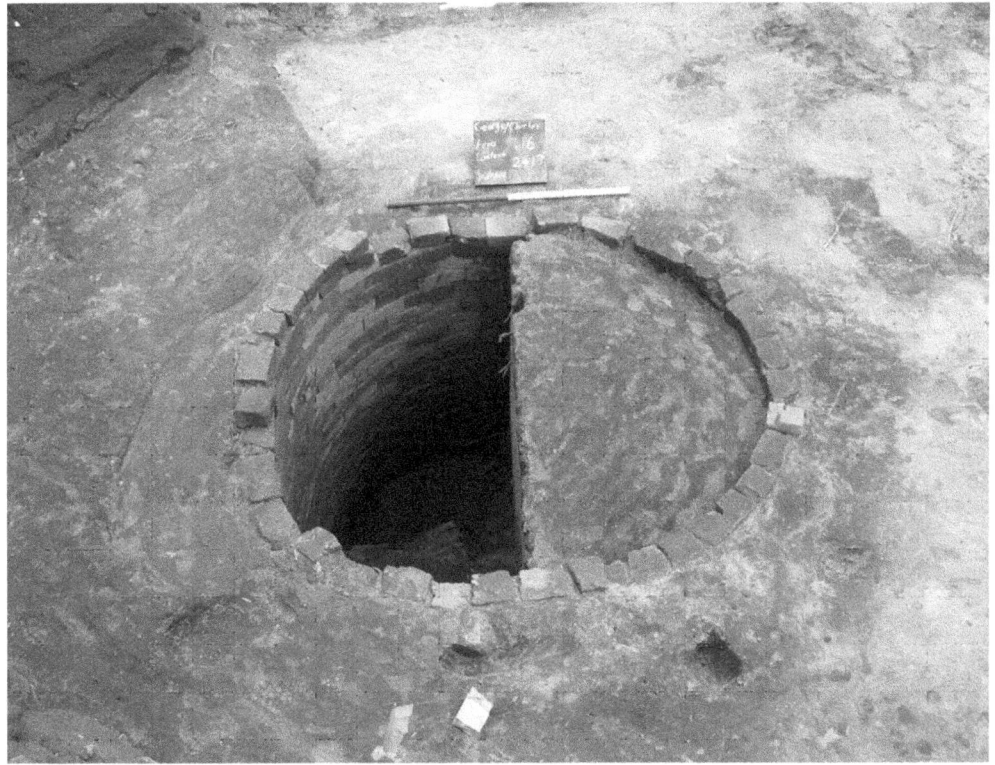

Figure A.10 Well (site 6). Allotment 69, 100 George Street, used in the case study. Source: Miskella 2003, 7.

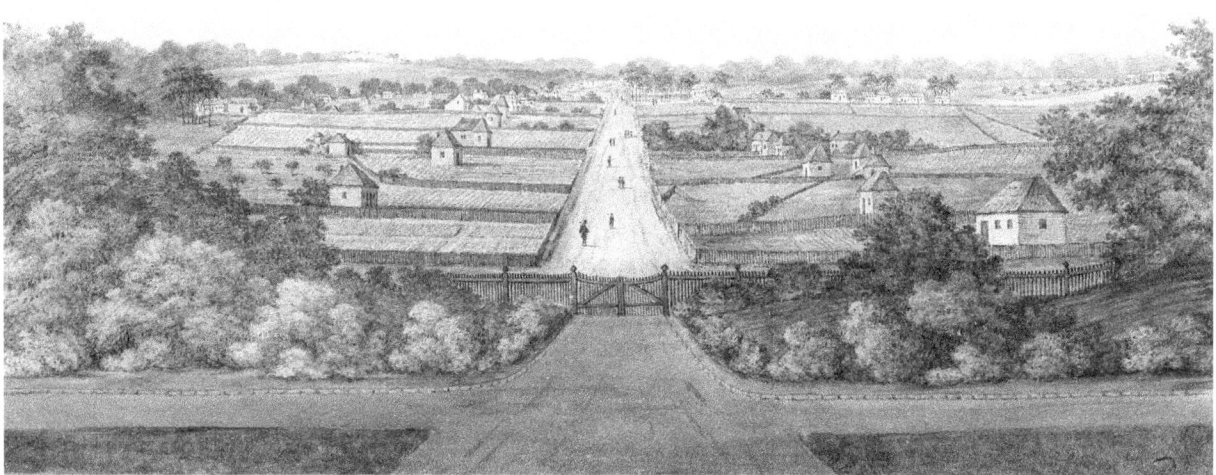

Figure A.11 An 1804–05 watercolour of convict huts along High Street (now George Street), Parramatta. Attributed to George Evans. Source: Courtesy the Caroline Simpson Collection, Historic Houses Trust of New South Wales, Museum of Sydney, MOS2007/15.

Site 7: 2 George Street

Lot 102 George Street (later 2 George Street) is located on a natural sandy slope near the corner of O'Connell Street and south of a natural creek. The first recorded occupant of 2 George Street was Anthony Landrin (né Antoine L'Andre), the liberated French prisoner-of-war sent to the colony in 1801 to establish viticulture for Governor King. In 1809 Landrin acquired the lease on the one-acre Lot 102 at what is now known as 2 George Street. An 1804–05 watercolour shows a view along George Street from Government House gates that includes 2 George Street with a convict hut and fruit trees (Figure A.11). Emancipated convict Samuel Larkin acquired the lease on the property in 1811 after Landrin's death, and by an 1824 account the convict hut was replaced with a weatherboarded and shingled house, and a garden well stocked with fruit trees.[7] Larkin is definitely known to have lived at this location from 1824 and in 1831 received his grant for the 1-acre property. Larkin's widow sold the property in 1838; subsequently, a brewery was constructed on the lot.[8]

Storage pits are common features identified during archaeological investigations of many convict hut sites, but brick-lined cellars with a tiled-roof timber superstructure are not.[9] An abandoned cellar (Context 3957) was located at the rear of Lot 102 (Figures A.12 and A.13). A total of 1,747 artefacts representing 457 MIC were recovered from this feature. The sandstock roofing tiles found in the demolition rubble indicate that the structure was constructed by 1810 and therefore was built by Anthony Landrin.[10] Approximately 84 per cent of the artefacts provided temporal data that were used to establish a 1790–1830 date range. This indicates the cellar was demolished and backfilled with mixed demolition debris and residential rubbish around the late 1830s, and the artefacts originated from the households of Landrin or Larkin, or both. While there were six distinct depositional episodes in the cellar, analysis results identified no discernible temporal difference in these deposits. There is slight contamination of data between deposits. A portion of this cellar was subject to a robbery attempt by a bottle collector and a cut for a 1950s service trench. This contamination was limited to a kiln tile from the 1850s brewery phase of site development and a patented 1885 aerated water bottle. Nevertheless, the stratified deposits are thought to be mixed, and the artefacts in these deposits are considered here as one.

---

7 *Sydney Gazette and New South Wales Advertiser* 15 April 1824, 1.
8 Higginbotham and Johnson 1989, 6–7.
9 Casey & Lowe 2006a, 60.
10 Stocks 2008, 32.

Appendix: sites in the case study

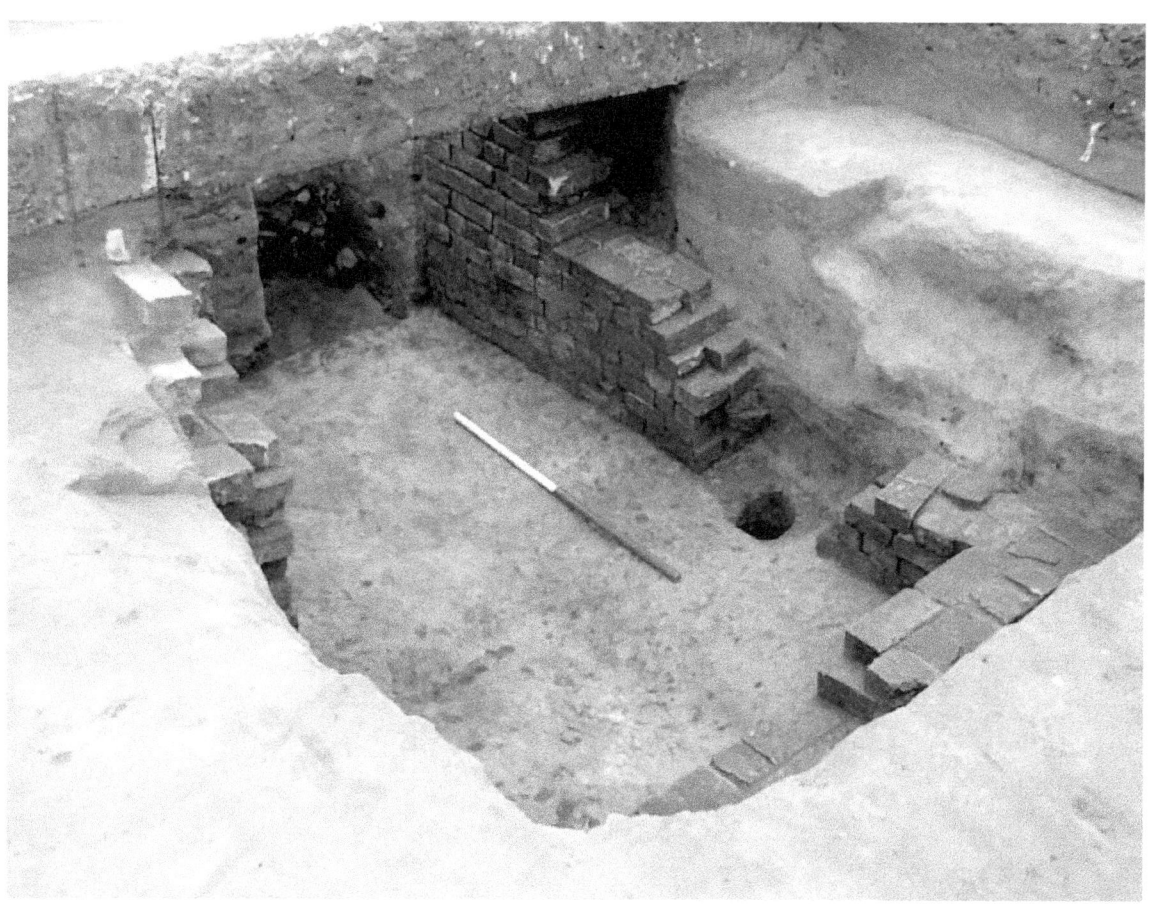

Figure A.12 Cellar at 2 George Street (site 7), used in the case study. Source: Casey & Lowe 2006a, 60.

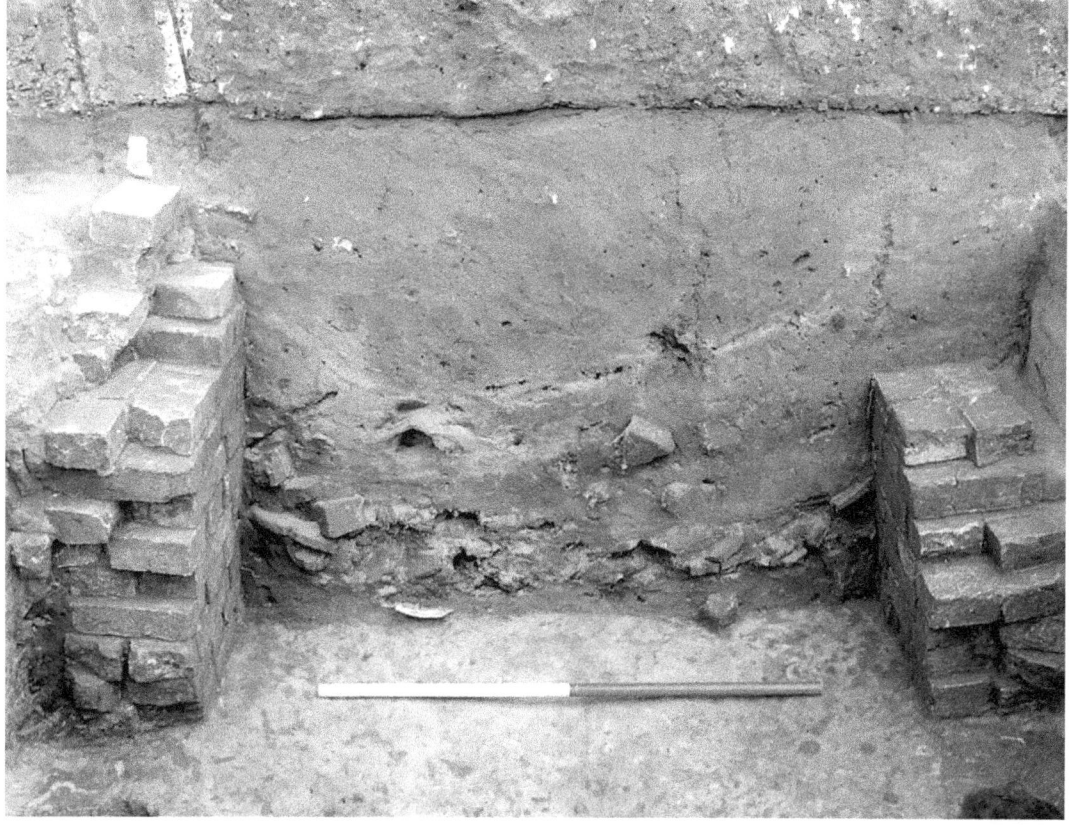

Figure A.13 Cellar profile at 2 George Street (site 7), used in the case study. Source: Casey & Lowe 2006a, 62.

Site 8: 109 George Street

In 1799, Rowland Hassall received a 14-year lease on a one-acre lot at what is now known as 109 George Street. The land was part of a natural alluvial terrace with a gentle slope to the Parramatta River. In 1804, Hassall's lease was converted to a land grant, and he built a brick home at 109 George Street. Within a few months, Hassall had informally acquired adjacent leases expanding his property to 5.5 acres. Over time the Hassall property became a well-developed complex including gardens and a dairy.[11]

Archaeological investigations excavated a series of pit cuts across the site. Based on the composition of the fill and results of pollen analysis, most pits were identified as compost pits rather than the anticipated rubbish pits. However, one pit (Context 5073) was filled with rubbish and temporal analysis of inclusive artefacts in the deposit indicate an 1820–1880 date range.[12] A total of 587 artefacts representing 248 MIC were recovered from this pit.

11　Binney 2005, 64.
12　Casey & Lowe 2006a, 94–5.

REFERENCES

Abercrombie, N. and B.S. Turner (1978). The dominant ideology thesis. *British Journal of Sociology* 29(2):149–70.

Accum, F. (1820). *Treatise on adulterations of food and culinary poisons.* St Louis, MO: Mallinckrodt Chemical Works.

Aird, W.V. (1961). *The water supply, sewerage and drainage of Sydney.* Sydney: Halstead Press.

Allen, Matthew (2011). Sectarianism, respectability and cultural identity: the St Patrick's Total Abstinence Society and Irish Catholic temperance in mid-19th century Sydney. *Journal of Religious History* 35(3): 374–92.

Bach, J. (1976). *A maritime history of Australia.* Sydney: Pan Books.

Baer, H.A., M. Singer and I. Susser (2003). *Medical anthropology and the world system.* London: Praeger.

Baker, P. and G. Carr (2002). *Practitioners, practices and patients: new approaches to medical archaeology and anthropology.* Proceedings of a conference held at Magdalene College, Cambridge.

Barton, G.B. (1989). *History of New South Wales from the records.* Sydney: Charles Potter, Government Printer.

Beasley, H. (1886). *The druggists general recipe book.* Philadelphia, PA: Lindsay & Blakiston.

Beaudry, M.C., L.J. Cook and S.A. Mrozowski (1991). Artifacts and active voices: material culture as social discourse. Originally published in R. McGuire and R. Paynter (eds), *The archaeology of inequality,* 150–291. Oxford: Blackwell Publishers.

Beaudry, M.C. and S. Mrozowski (1988). The archeology of work and home life in Lowell, Massachusetts: an interdisciplinary study of the Boott Cotton Mills Corporation. *Journal of the Society for Industrial Archeology* 2: 1–22.

Beeton, I. (1861). *Book of household management,* facsimile edn. New York: Farrar, Straus, & Giroux.

Benedict, R. (1934). *Patterns of culture.* Boston, MA: Houghton Mifflin.

Bennett, S. (1865). *The history of Australian discovery and colonisation.* Sydney: Hanson & Bennett.

Billen, G., J. Garnier, C. Deligne and C. Billen (1999). Estimates of early-industrial inputs of nutrients to river systems: implication for coastal eutrophication. *Science of the Total Environment* 243–244: 43–52. DOI: 10.1016/S0048-9697(99)00327-7.

Binney, K.R. (2005). *Horsemen of the first frontier (1788–1900) and the serpent's legacy.* Neutral Bay, NSW: Volcanic Productions.

Blainey, G. (2003). *Black kettle and full moon: daily life in a vanished Australia.* Melbourne: Viking Press.

Blainey, G. (1963). *The rush that never ended.* Melbourne: Melbourne University Press.

Blair, S. (1983). The felonry and the free? Divisions in the colonial society in the penal era. *Labour History* 45: 1–16.

Blocker, J.S., D.M. Fahey and I.R. Tyrrell (2003). *Alcohol and temperance in modern history: an international encyclopedia* volumes 1 and 2. Santa Barbara, CA: ABC-CLIO.

Bogle, M. (1993). *Vaucluse House.* Sydney: Historic House Trust of New South Wales.

Bonasera, M.C. (2001). Good for what ails you: medicinal use at Five Points. *Historical Archaeology* 35(3): 49–64.

Bongiorno, F. (2012). *The sex lives of Australians: a history.* Melbourne: Black Inc.

Brown, D.W. (1987). Muscular christianity in the Antipodes: some observations on the diffusion and emergence of a Victorian ideal in Australian social theory. *Journal of the Australian Society for Sports History* 3(2): 173–87.

Brown, K.M. (1937). *Medical practice in old Parramatta.* Sydney: Angus & Robertson.

Brown, P.J. and S. Closser (2016). *Understanding and applying medical anthropology.* London and New York: Routledge.

Brown, S. and K. Brown (1995). *Parramatta, a town caught in time, 1870.* Sydney: Hale & Iremonger.

Bulwer-Lytton, E. (1838). Paul Clifford. *A collection of ancient and modern British authors,* volume XLIX. Paris: Casimir.

Bushman, R.L. and C.L. Bushman (1988). The early history of cleanliness in America. *Journal of American History* 74(4): 1213–38.

Bynum, W.F. (1994). *Science and the practice of medicine in the 19th century.* Cambridge, UK: Cambridge University Press.

Campbell, R. (1983). The medical history of the Mint building. In J. Pearn and C. O'Carrigan (eds), *Australia's quest for colonial health*, 39–44. Brisbane: Department of Child Health, Royal Children's Hospital.

Campbell, W.S. (1932). The use and abuse of stimulants in the early days of settlement in New South Wales. *Journal of Royal Australian Historical Society* 18: 74–99.

Cannon, M. (1975). *Life in the cities*. Australia in the Victorian Age, volume 3. Melbourne: Thomas Nelson.

Cannon, M. (1971). *Who's master? Who's man?* Melbourne: Viking O'Neil.

Carpenter, M.W. (2010). *Health, medicine, and society in Victorian England*. Santa Barbara, CA: ABC-CLIO.

Carskadden, J. and R. Gartley 1990). A preliminary seriation of 19th-century decorated porcelain marbles. *Historical Archaeology* 24(2): 55–69.

Cartwright, F.F. (1972). *Disease and history*. New York: Thomas Y. Crowell.

Cavender, A. (2003). *Folk medicine in southern Appalachia*. Chapel Hill, NC: University of North Carolina Press.

Chase, K. (1991). *Middlemarch, landmarks of world literature*. Cambridge, UK: Cambridge University Press.

Clements, F. (1986). *A history of human nutrition in Australia*. Melbourne: Longman Cheshire.

Collins, D. (1798 [2003]). *An account of the English colony in New South Wales*, volume 1. Glasgow: Good Press.

Connell, R.W. and T.H. Irving (1980). *Class structure in Australian history*. Melbourne: Longman Cheshire.

Cook, K.E. (2008). *The Sage encyclopedia of qualitative research methods*, volume 2. Thousand Oaks, CA: Sagepub.

Cordery, S. (1995). Friendly societies and the discourse of respectability in Britain, 1825–1875. *Journal of British Studies* 34(1): 35–58.

Cowan, H.J. (1998). *From wattle and daub to concrete and steel: the engineering heritage of Australia's buildings*. Melbourne: Melbourne University Press.

Coward, D.H. (1988). *Out of sight: Sydney's environmental history 1851–1981*. Canberra: Australian National University.

Cressey, P. and J. Stephens (1982). The city-site approach to urban archaeology. In R. S. Dickens (ed.), *Archaeology of Urban America: the search for pattern and process*. Academic Press, New York.

Croft, J. (1999). A sense of industrial place: the literature of Newcastle, New South Wales, 1797–1997. *Antipodes* 13(1): 15–20.

Crook, P. and T. Murray (2004). The analysis of cesspit deposits from The Rocks, Sydney. *Australasian Journal of Historical Archaeology* 22: 44–56.

Davies, P. (2011). Destitute women and smoking at the Hyde Park Barracks, Sydney, Australia. *International Journal of Historical Archaeology* 15(1): 82–101.

Denny, N. (1988). Temperance and the Scottish churches,187–1914. *Scottish Church History Society,* 217–39.

Deutsher, K.M. (1999). *The breweries of Australia: a history*. Melbourne: Lothian Books.

Dillon, P. (2002). *Gin: the much-lamented death of Madam Geneva – The eighteen-century gin craze*. Boston, MA: Justin, Charles & Co.

Dingle, A.E. (1980). "The truly magnificent thirst": an historical survey of Australian drinking habits. *Historical Studies* 19: 227–49.

Dinneford & Co. (1854). *The family medicine directory*. Simpkin, Marshall & Co.

Donlon, D., M. Casey, W. Haak and C. Adler (2008). Early colonial burial practices for perinates at the Parramatta convict hospital, NSW. *Australasian Historical Archaeology* 26: 71–83.

Dyke, T. (2014). A history of health and medical research in Australia. *Medical Journal of Australia* 201(1). DOI: 10.5694/mja14.00347.

Eckersley, R. (2001). Culture, health and wellbeing. In R. Eckersley, J. Dixon and B. Douglas (eds), *Social Origins of Health and Well-being*. Cambridge, UK: Cambridge University Press.

Emmins, C. (1991). *Soft drinks and their origins*. London: Shire Publications Ltd.

Evans D. (1983). The plight of the poor in the working-man's paradise. In J. Pearn and C. O'Carrigan (eds), *Australia's quest for colonial health*, 203–12. Brisbane: Department of Child Health, Royal Children's Hospital.

Ferngren, G.B. (2014). *Medicine and religion: a historical introduction*. Baltimore, MD: Johns Hopkins University Press.

Fisher, C. and C. Kent (1999). *Two depressions, one banking collapse*. Research discussion paper. Sydney: System Stability Department, Reserve Bank of Australia.

Fisher, P. (2012). What is homeopathy? An introduction. *Frontiers in Bioscience* 4(5): 1669–82. DOI: 10.2741/489.

Fitts, R.K. (1999). The archaeology of middle-class domesticity and gentility in Victorian Brooklyn. *Historical Archaeology* 33(1): 39–62.

Flannery, T. (1999). *The birth of Sydney*. Melbourne: Text Publishing.

Foley, J.D. (1995). *In quarantine: a history of Sydney's Quarantine Station 1828–1984*. Sydney: Kangaroo Press.

Franklin, B. (1855). *Early rising, a natural social and religious duty*. Northhampton, UK: Abel & Sons.

Freeman, A.H. (n.d.) *The history of telephone switching technology in Australia: 1880–1980*. Australian Telecommunications monograph no. 5. Melbourne: Telecommunication Society of Australia.

Freeman, M. (2001). Oral hygiene: long in the tooth. *Chemist & Druggist* 22.

Fricker, J.P., M. Kiley, G. Townsend and C. Trevitt (2011). Professionalism: what is it, why should we have it and how can we achieve it? *Australian Dental Journal* 56: 92–6.

Gandevia, B. (1975). Socio-medical factors in the evolution of the First Settlement at Sydney Cove 1788–1803. *Royal Australian Historical Society* 61(1).

Gandevia, B. (1978). *Tears often shed: child health and welfare in Australia from 1788*. Sydney: Pergamon Press.

Garton, S. (1990). *Out of luck: poor Australians and social welfare*. Sydney: Allen & Unwin,

Gibbs, M. (2012). The convict system of New South Wales: a review of archaeological research since 2001. *Archaeology in Oceania* 47(2): 78–83.

Gillen, M. (1989). *The founders of Australia: a biographical dictionary of the First Fleet*. Sydney: Library of Australian History.

Gojak, D. and I. Stuart (1999). The potential for the archaeological study of clay tobacco pipes from Australian sites. *Australasian Historical Archaeology* 17: 38–49.

Graham, K. (2005). The archaeological potential of medicinal advertisements. *Australasian Historical Archaeology* 23: 47–53.

Green, D. and L. Cromwell (1984). *Mutual aid or welfare state: Australia's friendly societies*. Sydney: Allen & Unwin.

Grehan, M. (2009). Heroes or villains? Midwives, nurses, and maternity care in mid-19th century Australia. *Traffic* 11: 55–72.

Griggs, P. (2011). *Global industry, local innovation: the history of cane sugar production in Australia, 1820–1995*. Bern, Switzerland: Peter, Lange.

Gusfield, J.R. (1986). *Symbolic crusade: status politics and the American temperance movement*. Champaign, IL: University of Illinois Press.

Hagger, J. (1979). *Australian colonial medicine*. Adelaide: Rigby Ltd.

Haley, B. (1979). *The healthy body and Victorian culture*. Cambridge, MA: Harvard University Press.

Hands, T. (2018). *Drinking in Victorian and Edwardian Britain: beyond the spectre of the drunkard*. Palgrave Macmillan (ebook).

Harol C. (2006). Introduction: virginity and patrilinear legitimacy. In *Enlightened virginity in 18th-century literature*. New York: Palgrave Macmillan.

Harris, E.J. (2019). Health concerns and remedies in 19th-century Parramatta: a look at patent and proprietary medicine. *Australasian Historical Archaeology* 37: 26–36.

Harris, E.J., G. Ginn and C. Coroneous (2004). How to dig a dump: strategy and research design for investigation of Brisbane's 19th-century municipal dump. *Australasian Historical Archaeology* 20: 15–26.

Harris, J. and I. Smith (2005). The Te Hoe Shore Whaling Station artefact assemblage. *Otago Archaeological Laboratory Report: Number 2*. Otago, New Zealand: University of Otago.

Hartz, L. (1964). *The founding of new societies: studies in the history of the United States, Latin America, South Africa, Canada and Australia*. New York: Harcourt Brace & World.

Hassam, A. (1994). *Sailing to Australia: shipboard diaries by 19th-century British emigrants*. Manchester, UK: Manchester University Press.

Hassell, Reverend J.S. (1902). *In old Australia*. Brisbane: R.S. Hews & Co.

Hayes, S. (2014). *Good taste, fashion, luxury: A genteel Melbourne family and their rubbish*. Sydney: Sydney University Press.

Hendriksen, G. and C. Liston, eds (2008). *Woman transported: life in Australia's convict female factories*. Parramatta, NSW: Parramatta Heritage Centre.

Herman, M. (1970). *The early Australian architects and their work*. Sydney: Angus & Robertson.

Henry, F.J.J. (1939). *New South Wales. Metropolitan Water*. Sydney: Sewerage and Drainage Board, Sydney Water Department.

Higginbotham, E. (1983). The excavation of a brick barrel-drain at Parramatta, N.S.W. *Australian Historical Archaeology* 1: 35–9.

Hirst, J. (2009). *Sense and nonsense in Australian history*. Melbourne: Black Inc.

Historic Houses Trust of New South Wales (1995). *Elizabeth Farm Parramatta: a history and a guide*. Sydney: Historic Houses Trust of New South Wales.

Horton, D. (1943). The function of alcohol in primitive societies: A cross cultural study. *Quarterly Journal of Studies of Alcohol* 4: 199–320.

Hsu, E. (2000). Medical anthropology, material culture, and new directions in medical archaeology. In P. Baker and G. Carr (eds), *Practitioners, practices and patients: new approaches to medical archaeology and anthropology*. Oxford, UK: Oxbow Books.

Hubbard, G.H., ed. (1853 [2011]). *New Hampshire Journal of Medicine*. Michigan, IL: University of Michigan.

Hughes, R. (1986). *The fatal shore: the epic of Australia's founding*. New York: Random House.

Hughes, T. (1880). *Tom Brown at Oxford*. London: Porter & Coates.

Huneman, P. (2008). Montpellier vitalism and the emergence of alienism in France (1750–1800): the case of passions. *Science in Context* 21(4): 615–47. DOI: 10.1017/s0269889708001981.

Iacono, N. (2002). Beyond the breach: advancing strategies for archaeological management plans. *Australasian Historical Archaeology* 20: 39–47.

Jackson, L. (2014). *Dirty old London: the Victorian fight against filth*. New Haven, CT: Yale University Press.

James, S. (2010). Farming on the fringe: peri-urban market gardens within Sydney's historical and contemporary cityscape. *Greenfields, brownfields, newfields: 10th Urban History Planning Conference*, Melbourne.

Jamison, T. (1804). General observation on the small pox. *Sydney Gazette and New South Wales Advertiser*, 14 October, 2.

Jervis, J. (1963). *The cradle city of Australia: a history of Parramatta 1788–1961*. Parramatta, NSW: Council of the City of Parramatta.

Johnson, M. (2010). *Archaeological theory: an introduction*. Chichester, UK: Wiley-Blackwell.

Jones, D. (2009). *Thirsty work, the story of Sydney's soft drink manufacturers*. Glebe, NSW: David V. Jones.

Kass, T., C. Liston and J. McClymont (1996). *Parramatta: a past revealed*. Parramatta, NSW: Parramatta City Council.

Karamanou, M., G. Panayiotakopoulos, G. Tsoucalas, A.A. Kousoulis and G. Androutso (2012). From miasmas to germs: a historical approach to theories of infectious disease transmission. *Le Infezioni in Medicina* 1: 52–6.

Karskens, G. (2010). *The colony: a history of early Sydney*. Sydney: Allen & Unwin.

Keating, P. J. (1971). *The working classes in Victorian fiction*. London: Routledge & Kegan Paul.

Keneally, T. (2006). *Commonwealth of thieves*. Sydney: Random House Australia.

Kimber, J. and P. Love (2001). The time of their lives. In *The Time of Their Lives; The eight hour day and working life*. Broadway, NSW: Australian Society for Study of Labour History.

Kingsley, H. (1860). *The recollections of Geoffrey Hamlyn*. Cambridge, UK: Cambridge University Press.

Kottaras, P. (2009). 150 Marsden Street. In *Breaking the Shackles*. Parramatta, NSW: A Parramatta Heritage Centre and Casey & Lowe Pty Ltd publication.

Larcombe, F.A. (1973). *The origin of local government in New South Wales 1858–1906*. Sydney: Sydney University Press.

Lawrence, S. and P. Davies (2010). *An archaeology of Australia since 1788*. Berlin: Springer Science & Business Media (ebook).

LeeDecker, C.H. (1991). Historical dimensions of consumer research. In T. Klein and C. LeeDecker (eds), *Models for the study of consumer behaviour. Historical Archaeology* Special Issue 25(2): 30–45.

Levine, W.S. (1996). *The control handbook*. Boca Raton, FL: CRC Press (ebook).

Lewis, M. (2014). Medicine in colonial Australia 1788–1900. *Medical Journal of Australia* 201(1): S5–S10.

Lewis, M. (1992). *A rum state: alcohol and state policy in Australia 1788–1988*. Canberra: Australian Government Publishing Service.

References

Lewis, M.J. (2003). *The people's heath: public health in Australia 1788–1950*. London: Praeger.

Little, B.J. (1994). People with history: an update on historical archaeology in the United States. *Journal of Archaeological Method and Theory* 1(1): 1–40.

Loddenkemper, R. and M. Kreuter (2015). *The tobacco epidemic*. Basel, Switzerland: S. Karger AG (ebook).

Loomis, C.G. (1949). Indications of miners' medicine. *Western Folklore* 8: 117–22.

Lydon, J. (1993). Archaeology in The Rocks, Sydney, 1979–1993: from Old Sydney Gaol to Mrs Lewis' boardinghouse. *Australasian Historical Archaeology* 11: 33–41.

MacPhail, M. and M. Casey (2008). "News from the interior": what can we tell from plant microfossils preserved on historical archaeological sites in colonial Parramatta? *Australasian Historical Archaeology* 26: 45–69.

Mann, D.D. (1979). *The present picture of New South Wales*, 2nd edn. Sydney: John Ferguson.

Mant, M. and C. Roberts (2014). Diet and dental caries in post-medieval London. *International Journal of Historical Archaeology* 19: 188–207.

Marsden, J.B., ed. (1858 [2010]). *Memoirs of the life and labours of Rev. Samuel Marsden of Parramatta, senior chaplin of New South Wales; and of his early connexion with the missions of New Zealand and Tahiti*. London: Religious Tract Society (ebook).

Marsh, M. (1990). *Suburban lives*. New Brunswick, NJ: Rutgers University Press.

Martyr, P. (2002). *Paradise of Quacks: an alternative history of medicine in Australia*. Sydney: Macleay Press.

Mattick, B.E. (2010). *A guide to bone toothbrushes of the 19th and early 20th centuries*. Bloomington, IN: Xlibris.

Mauriceau, A.M. (1855 [1984]). *The married woman's private medical companion*. New York: Arno Press.

Maxwell-Stewart, H.J. (2006). Crime and health: an introductory overview. In P.A.C. Richards (ed), *Effecting a cure: aspects of health and medicine in Launceston*, 35–54. Launceston, TAS: Myola House of Publishing.

McMichael, P. (1980). Crisis in pastoral capital accumulation: a re-interpretation of the 1840s depression in colonial Australia. *Essays in the Political Economy of Australian Capitalism*, volume 4, 17–40. Sydney: Australia & New Zealand Book Co.

McNulty, R.H. (2004). *Dutch glass bottles of the 17th and 18th centuries*. Bethesda, MD: Medici Workshop.

Miller, D. (1995). *Acknowledging consumption*. London: Routledge.

Miller, H. (1988). Baroque cities in the wilderness: archaeology and urban development in the colonial Chesapeake. *Historical Archaeology* 22(2): 57–73.

Miss Leslie (1864). *The ladies' guide to true politeness and perfect manners or, Miss Leslie's behaviour book*. Philadelphia, PA: T.B. Peterson & Brothers.

Mitchell, S. (1981). *The fallen angels: chastity, class, and women's readings 1835–1880*. Wisconsin: Popular Press.

Mrozowski, S. (2006). *The archaeology of class in urban America*. Cambridge, UK: Cambridge University Press.

Murdock, C.G. (1998). *Domesticating drink: women, men, and alcohol in America, 1870–1940*. Baltimore, MD: Johns Hopkins University Press.

Mwinyihija, M. (2010). *Ecotoxicological diagnosis in the tanning industry*. Springer (ebook).

New South Wales Health Department (1997). One hundred years of vaccination. *NSW Public Health Bulletin* 8(8–9): 61–3.

Office of Minister of Public Health (1903). Register of Dentists of the State of New South Wales, as printed in the *Government Gazette of New South Wales for 1902*, 6 February 1903, 1049.

Oxley, D. (1996). *Convict maids: the forced migration of women to Australia*. Cambridge, UK: Cambridge University Press.

Paul, J.R. and P.W. Parmalee (1973). *Soft drink bottling*. Springfield, IL: Illinois State Museum Society.

Pearce, J.M.S. (2003). Historical note – Sir Thomas Clifford Allbutt. *Journal of Neurology, Neurosurgery and Psychiatry* 74: 1443.

People's Publishing Company (1885 [1980]). *Australian Etiquette, or the rules and usages of the best society in the Australian colonies*, facsimile edn. Melbourne: J.M. Dent.

Peterkin, A. (2001). *One thousand beards: a cultural history of facial hair*. Vancouver, BC: Arsenal Pulp Press.

Peterson, J. (1979). The impact of sanitary reform upon American urban planning 1840–1890. *Journal of Social History* 13(1): 83–103.

Piddock, S. (2007). *A space of their own: the archaeology of 19th century lunatic asylums in Britain, South Australia and Tasmania.* New York: Springer (ebook).

Pirhonen, I., A. Nevalainen, T. Husman and J. Pekkanen (1996). Home dampness, moulds and their influences on respiratory infections and symptoms in adults in Finland. *European Respiratory Journal*: 2618–22.

Polya, R. (2001). *Food regulation in Australia – a chronology.* Canberra: Department of the Parliamentary Library.

Porter, R. (1993). *Disease, medicine and society in England, 1550–1860.* Cambridge, UK: Cambridge University Press.

Porter, R. (1982). *English society in the 18th century.* Harmondsworth, UK: Pelican Books.

Potter, L. (2017). *Mistress of her profession: colonial midwives of Sydney, 1788–1901.* Sydney: Anchor Books.

Prester, L. (2011). Indoor exposure to mould allergens. *Industrial Hygiene and Toxicology* 62(4): 371–80.

Priestley, J. (1772). *Directions for impregnating water with fixed air; in order to communicate to it the peculiar spirit and virtues of Pyrmont water, and other mineral waters of a similar nature.* London: Printed for J. Johnson.

Proudfoot, H. (1988). Fixing the settlement upon a savage shore: planning and building. In G. Aplin (ed.), *Sydney before Macquarie: a difficult infant,* 72–91. Sydney: New South Wales University Press.

Quirk, K. (2008). The colonial goldfields: vision and revisions. *Australasian Historical Archaeology* 26: 13–20.

Reckner, P.E. and S.A. Brighton (1999). Free from all vicious habits. *Historical Archaeology* 33(1): 63–86.

Reese, J. (1991). *Index: Female Factory Parramatta 1826 to 1848.* Compiled from primary records with kind permission of the Archives Office of New South Wales (microfiche).

Richards, D. (1987). Transported to New South Wales: medical convicts 1788–1850. *British Medical Journal* 295: 1603–12.

Richards, E. (1993). *How did the poor emigrate from the British Isles to Australia in the 19th century?* Canberra: Australia National University.

Richards, M., H. Hyde and D.A. Williams (1956). Allergy to mould spores in Britain. *British Medical Journal* 1(4972): 886–90.

Ritter, T.J. (1917). *Mother's remedies: over one thousand tried and tested remedies from mothers of the United States and Canada,* rev. edn. Detroit, MI: G.H. Foote.

Rivett, C. (1961). *An artist's guide to old Parramatta.* Sydney: H.H. Dowling.

Roberts, D. (2011). The "knotted hands that set us high": labour history and the study of convict Australia. *Labour History* (100): 33–50.

Roche, A.M., P. Bywood, T. Freeman, K. Pidd, J. Borlagdan and A. Trifonoff (2009). *The social context of alcohol use in Australia.* Adelaide: National Centre for Education and Training on Addiction.

Roe, J. (1975). Social policy and the permanent poor. In E.L. Wheelwright and K. Buckley (eds), *The political economy of Australian capitalism,* 82–4. Sydney: Australia & New Zealand Book Co.

Rosecrance, R.N. (1964). The radical culture of Australia. In L. Hartz, ed. *The founding of new societies,* 275–318, New York: Harcourt, Brace & World, Inc. (Kindle ebook).

Rosecrance, R.N. (1960). The radical tradition in Australia: an interpretation. *Review of Politics,* 22(1): 115–32.

Rosenthal, J. (2019). *Good form: the ethical experience of the Victorian novel.* Princeton, NJ: Princeton University Press.

Sands, J. (1931). *Sands Sydney & Suburban Directory 1931.* Sydney: Robert Sands.

Salt, A. (1984). *These outcast women: the Parramatta Female Factory 1821–1848.* Sydney: Hale & Iremonger.

Schiffer, M.B. (1987). *Formation processes of the archaeological record.* Albuquerque, NM: University of New Mexico.

Shanks, M. (2007). Post-processual archaeology and after. In R. Alexander Bentley, H.D.G. Maschner and C. Chippindale, (eds), *Handbook of archaeological theories,* 133–43. Lanham, MD: AltaMira Press.

Shann, E. (1930). *An economic history of Australia.* Melbourne: Georgian House.

Shinman, L.L. (1972). The Church of England Temperance Society in the 19th century. *Historical Magazine of the Protestant Episcopal Church* 41(2): 179–95.

Singer, M. and H. Baer (2012). *Introducing medical anthropology: a discipline in action.* Plymouth UK: Rowman & Littlefield Publishers.

Skinner, H.B. (1849). *The female's medical guide and married woman's adviser.* Boston, MA: self published.

Smith, F.H. (2008). *The archaeology of alcohol and drinking*. Gainesville FL: University Press of Florida.

Smith, J.C., H. Whiley and K.E. Ross (2021). The new environmental health in Australia: failure to launch? *International Journal of Environmental Research and Public Health* 18(4): 1402. DOI: 10.3390/ijerph18041402.

Smith, V. (2007). *Clean: a history of personal hygiene and purity*. Oxford, UK: Oxford University Press.

Stocks, R. (2008). New evidence for local manufacture of artefacts at Parramatta 1790–1830. *Australasian Historical Archaeology* 26: 29–43.

Sturma, M. (1983). *Vice in a vicious society*. Brisbane: University of Queensland Press.

Taylor, C. (2004). *Modern social imaginaries*. Durham, NC: Duke University Press.

Tench, W. (1793a [1979]). *Sydney's first four years*, ed. L.F. Fitzhardinge. Sydney: Library of Australian History.

Tench, W. (1793b [1988]). *A complete account of the settlement at Port Jackson; including an accurate description of the situation of the colony; of the natives; and of its natural production*, digitised text sponsored by University of Sydney Library (ebook).

Terry, L. (2013). Caboonbah: the archaeology of a middle class Queensland pastoral family. *International Journal of Historical Archaeology* 17(3): 569–89.

Therry, R. (1863). *Reminiscences of thirty years' residence in New South Wales and Victoria*. London: Sampson Low, Son & Co.

Toffler, A. (1970). *Future Shock*. London: Bodley Head.

Towler, J. and J. Bramall (1986). *Midwives in history and society*. Sydney: Croom Helm.

Tyrrell, I. (2008). From the culture of wowserism to the culture of healthism: law, custom, fashion and etiquette in Australian smoking,1900–1990s. Paper presented at the Virtues of Self-Control and Moderation conference. University of New South Wales, 8 December.

Valuck, R.J., S. Poirier and R.G. Mrtek (1992). Patent medicine muckraking: influences on American pharmacy, social reform and foreign authors. *Pharmacy in History* 34(4): 183–292.

Walker, R. (1984). *Under fire: a history of tobacco smoking in Australia*. Melbourne: Melbourne University Press.

Walker, R.B. (1980). Medical aspects of tobacco smoking and anti-tobacco movement in Britain in the 19th century. *Medical History* 24(4): 391–402.

Watson, N.J., S. Weir and S. Friend (2005). The development of muscular Christianity in Victorian Britain and beyond, *Journal of Religion and Society* 7:1–17.

Wear, A. (2000). *Knowledge and practice in English medicine 1550–1680*. Cambridge, UK: Cambridge University Press.

Webb, A.D. (1913). The consumption of alcoholic liquors in the United Kingdom. *Journal of the Royal Statistical Society* 76(2): 207–20.

Wesleyan Methodist Connection (1843). *Discipline of the Wesleyan Methodist Church of America*. Boston, MA: O. Scott.

Wharton, J.C. (1911). *The jubilee history of Parramatta*. Parramatta, NSW: Cumberland Argus Printing Works.

Wheeler, K. (2000). Theoretical and methodological considerations for excavating privies. *Historical Archaeology* 34(1): 3–19.

Wilson, G.B. (1940). *Alcohol and the nation: a contribution to the study of the liquor problem in the United Kingdom from 1800 to 1935*. London: Nicholson & Watson.

Witeska-Młynarczyk, A. (2012). Why and how to include anthropological perspective into multidisciplinary research in the Polish health system. *Annals of Agricultural and Environmental Medicine* 19(3): 497–501.

Woolsey, S.C. (1908). *The letters of Jane Austen*. Boston, MA: Little, Brown and Company.

World Health Organization (1978). *Primary health care*. Geneva, Switzerland: WHO.

Wright, C. (2003). *Beyond the ladies lounge: Australia's female publicans*. Melbourne: Melbourne University Press.

Wright, E.O. (2015). *Understanding class*. London: Verso.

Young, L. (1988). *Middle-class culture in the 19th century: America, Australia and Britain*. Basingstoke, UK: Palgrave Macmillan.

Youssef, H. (1993). The history of the condom. *Journal of Royal Society of Medicine* 86: 226.

Zierden, M. and E. Reitz (2016). *Charleston: an archaeology of life in a coastal community*. Gainesville, FL: University of Florida Press.

Unpublished source material – reports

Artefact Heritage (2019). Sydney Gateway Road Project: Environmental Impact Statement, Statement of Heritage impact. Prepared for Gateway to Sydney Joint Venture for Roads and Maritime Service.

Brown, A.G. and Ho Chin Ko (1997). Black wattle and its utilization. Prepared for Rural Industries Research and Development Corporation.

Carney, M. (1996). Woolcott's Dispensary 41–47 George Street. Prepared for Richardson & Wrench Pty Ltd and Siblow Pty Ltd.

Casey, M. (2005). Preliminary results, archaeological investigation, stage 1, Parramatta Hospital Site, Marsden & George streets, Parramatta. Prepared by Casey & Lowe Pty Ltd for New South Wales Department of Commerce, Sydney.

Casey & Lowe (2018). Parramatta North Growth Centre (PNGC), Cumberland Hospital (East Campus) Site & Norma Parker Centre/Kamballa Site. Report to UrbanGrowth NSW Development Corporation.

Casey & Lowe (2014). Baseline Archaeological Assessment & Statement of Heritage Impact: Historical Archaeology, Cumberland Precinct and Sport & Leisure Precinct, Parramatta North Urban Renewal–Rezoning. Report to UrbanGrowth NSW.

Casey & Lowe (2012). Archaeological investigations: 15 Macquarie Street, Parramatta. Report to Comber Consultants on behalf of Endeavour Energy.

Casey & Lowe (2006a). Archaeological investigation 109–113 George Street, Parramatta. Submitted to Landcom.

Casey & Lowe (2006b). Archaeological Investigation: Parramatta Children's Court, cnr George & O'Connell Street, Parramatta. Submitted to New South Wales Department of Commerce and New South Wales Attorney General's Department.

Casey & Lowe (2005a). Archaeological investigation, non-Indigenous archaeology, 1 Smith Street, Parramatta.

Casey & Lowe (2005b). Preliminary excavation, stage 2b – Blood Bank, Parramatta Justice Precinct, former Parramatta Hospital Site, George & Marsden streets, Parramatta. Prepared for Multiplex on behalf of the NSW Commerce Department.

Dusting, A. (2017). 8 Parramatta Square (8PS), 160–180 Church Street Parramatta. Casey & Lowe Pty Ltd, prepared for Walker Corporation.

Dusting, A. (2016). Parramatta Square PS3, 153 Macquarie Street, Parramatta. Preliminary results of the historical archaeological investigation, Casey & Lowe Pty Ltd. Report to Parramatta City Council.

Edward Higginbotham & Associates (2007). Report on the archaeological excavations, 134–140 Marsden Street & 45–47 Macquarie Street, Parramatta, N.S.W.

GML Heritage (2015). 143–169 Macquarie Street (One PSQ), Parramatta: historical archaeological excavation report. Prepared for Leighton Properties, Sydney.

Godden Mackay Logan (2000). Parramatta Historical Archaeological Landscape Management Study (PHALMS). Prepared for the New South Wales Heritage Office.

Green, A. and W. Thorp (1987). St Marys industrial heritage study. Prepared for Penrith City Council.

Harris, E.J. (2019). Glass report: 8PS 140–160 Church Street, Parramatta NSW. Prepared for Casey & Lowe Pty Ltd.

Harris, E.J. (2016). 161–165 Clarence Street & 304 Kent Street, Sydney, NSW 2000: analysis of artefacts. Prepared for E.A. Higginbotham and Associates, Sydney.

Harris, E.J. (2013). UniSA City West Learning Centre site: analysis of artefacts. Prepared for Austral Archaeology.

Harris, E.J (2010). Glass report: 710–722 George Street, Sydney City. Prepared for Casey & Lowe Pty Ltd.

Harris, E.J. (2007). Old Marulan 2007 archaeological investigation artefact analysis. Prepared for Banksia Heritage + Archaeology and Umwelt.

Harris, E.J. (2005). Specialist glass report: Red Cow Inn and Penrith Plaza, Penrith. Prepared for Casey & Lowe Pty Ltd, Leichhardt.

Higginbotham, E. (2007). Report on archaeological excavations, 134–140 Marsden Street and 45–47 Macquarie Street, Parramatta N.S.W. Vol. 2. Submitted to Estates Construction of Australia.

Higginbotham, E. (2004). Historical and archaeological assessment of a brick drain, Grose & Fennell streets, North Parramatta, N.S.W.

Higginbotham, E. (1981). The excavation of a brick-barrel drain at Parramatta, NSW. Report commissioned by the G.I.O. and presented to the Heritage Council of N.S.W.

Higginbotham, E. and P.A. Johnson (1989). The future of Parramatta's past. An archaeological zoning plan. 1788 to 1844. Vol. 1. University of New South Wales, and the Department of Planning, 19QO.

Kass, T. (2002). The history of a site in George and Charles streets Parramatta. Submitted to Casey & Lowe Pty Ltd.

Lawrie, R. (1981). Geology and topography in *The Excavation of a Brick Barrel Drain at Parramatta, N.S.W*. Prepared for the Heritage Council N.S.W.

Miskella, J. (2017). 8PS–Church Street Parramatta: Trench report, Area R, Lot 19 and 20. Prepared by Casey & Lowe Pty Ltd.

Miskella, J. (2005). Trench report: Lot 99 Stage 2b, rear of Blood Bank, Parramatta Justice Precinct. Prepared for Casey & Lowe Pty Ltd.

Miskella, J. (2003a). Trench report: Lot 70 George and Charles streets, Parramatta. Unpublished document prepared as part archaeological investigations, George and Charles streets, Parramatta (in preparation). Prepared by Casey & Lowe Pty Ltd.

Miskella, J. (2003b). Trench report: Lot 69 George and Charles streets, Parramatta. Unpublished document prepared as part archaeological investigations, George and Charles streets, Parramatta (in preparation), prepared by Casey & Lowe Pty Ltd.

Stocks, R. (2009). Miscellaneous, metals and organics report: Parramatta Hospital Site, Marsden and George streets, Parramatta. Prepared for Casey & Lowe Pty Ltd, Sydney.

Unpublished source material – theses

Allen, M. (2013). The temporal shift: drunkenness, responsibility and the regulation of alcohol in New South Wales, 1788–1856. PhD thesis, University of Sydney, Sydney.

Briggs, S. (2006). Portonian respectability: working-class attitudes to respectability in Port Adelaide through material culture 1840–1900. PhD thesis, Department of Archaeology, Flinders University of South Australia, Adelaide.

Crook, P. (2008). Superior quality: exploring the nature of cost, quality and value in historical archaeology. PhD thesis, La Trobe University, Melbourne.

de Looper, M.W. (2014). Death registration and mortality trends in Australia 1856–1906. PhD thesis, Australian National University, Canberra.

Elliot, J. (1988). The colonies clothed. PhD thesis, Department of History, University of Adelaide, Adelaide.

Forbes, P. (2016). The pleasure grounds of the Illawarra suburbs: early tourism on the Georges River, a dissertation submitted for the award of a Bachelor of Arts (Archaeology) Honours, University of New England.

Harris, E.J. (2021). Cleanliness is next to godliness: the influence of Victorian values on health concerns in nineteenth-century Parramatta NSW, a dissertation submitted to the University of New South Wales for the award of a Doctorate of Philosophy in Archaeology.

Johns, L. (2001). Women in colonial commerce 1817–1820: the window of understanding provided by the Bank of New South Wales ledger and minute books. Master's thesis, Australian National University, Canberra.

Jones, W.H. (2001). Jewish ritual washing and Christian baptism. Master's thesis, McMasters Divinity College, Hamilton, Ontario, Canada.

Longhurst, P. (2011). The foundations of madness: the role of built environment in mental institutions of New South Wales. BA (Hons) thesis, Department of Archaeology, University of Sydney, Sydney.

Lun, P. (2015). Of cures and nostrums: medicine and public health in Market Street Chinatown. PhD thesis, Department of Anthropology, Stanford University, Standford, CA.

Matheuszik, D.L. (2013). The angel paradox: Elizabeth Fry and the role of gender and religion in 19th-century Britain. PhD thesis, Department of History, Vanderbilt University, Nashville, TN.

Merritt, A.S. (1981). The development and application of masters and servants legislation in New South Wales –1845 to 1930. PhD thesis, Australian National University, Canberra.

Parker, M. (2006). Rethinking the convict huts of Parramatta: an archaeology of transformation (1790–1841). BA (Hons) thesis, Department of Archaeology, School of Philosophical and Historical Inquiry, University of Sydney, Sydney.

Sprenger, N.H. (2012). Health appropriation: a comparative study of patent medicines and orthodox medical practice, using colonial Queensland as a case study. PhD thesis, School of Social Science, University of Queensland, Brisbane.

Watson, C. (2018). Archaeology and temperance: measuring a century of household alcohol consumption in New Zealand. Master's thesis, University of Otago, Dunedin, New Zealand.

Internet sources

Australian Bureau of Statistics (2014). Australian historical population statistics. 3105.0.65.001. http://www.abs.gov.au/AUSSTATS/abs@.nsf/DetailsPage/3105.0.65.0012014?OpenDocument.

Australian Cane Farmers Association (2006). Historic events. https://www.acfa.com.au/sugar-industry/historical-events/.

Australian Government Bureau of Meteorology (n.d.) Climate statistics for Australian locations. http://www.bom.gov.au/climate/averages/tables/cw_066124.shtml.

Barker, G. (2015). The Old Markets in Parramatta Square 1813–1880. Parramatta Heritage Centre, Research Services. https://historyandheritage.cityofparramatta.nsw.gov.au/blog/2016/04/17/the-old-markets-in-parramatta-square-1813-1880.

Cameron, M. (2015). The Colonial Hospital. *Dictionary of Sydney*. https://dictionaryofsydney.org/place/parramatta.

Decker, E. (n.d.). A history of childrens tea sets. http://www.childs-tea-set.com/child-tea-set-history.htm.

Department of the Environment and Energy (n.d.). History – Parramatta Female Factory Precinct. Australian Government. https://www.environment.gov.au/system/files/consultations/b7d99d0f-dc3d-454b-9ac3-fa157f34cc83/files/

Due, S. (n.d.). *Australian medical pioneers index*. http://www.medicalpioneers.com/.

Dyster, B. (2022). The Depression of the 1840s in New South Wales. *Australian Dictionary of Biography*. National Centre of Biography, Australian National University. https://adb.anu.edu.au/essay/29/text40594.

Fitzgerald, S. (2008). Royal Commission on Noxious and Offensive Trades 1882. *Dictionary of Sydney*. https://dictionaryofsydney.org/entry/royal_commission_into_noxious_and_offensive_trades_1882.

Gilbert, L.A. (1966) Considen, Dennis (?–1815). *Australian Dictionary of Biography*. National Centre of Biography, Australian National University. http://adb.anu.edu.au/biography/considen-dennis-1916/text2277.

Gunson, N. (1966). Rowland Hassall (1768–1820). *Australian Dictionary of Biography*. National Centre of Biography, Australian National University. http://adb.anu.edu.au/biography/hassall-rowland-2166.

Homan, P.G. (2006). Daffy: a legend in his own preparation. *Pharmaceutical Journal*, 30 December. http://www.pharmaceutical-journal.com/opinion/comment/daffy-a-legend-in-his-own-preparation/10002899.article.

Lindsey, B. (2010). *Historic glass bottle identification and information website*. Society for Historical Archaeology and Bureau of Land Management. http://www.sha.org/bottle/index.htm.

McClymont, J. (2014). Thomas Halfpenny – George (High) Street – Parramatta Pioneers. Parramatta Heritage Centre. http://arc.parracity.nsw.gov.au/blog/2014/10/08/thomas-halfpenny-george-high-street-parramatta-pion.

McClymont, J. (1999). The new hospital for Parramatta. https://historyandheritage.cityofparramatta.nsw.gov.au/blog/2018/07/20/the-parramatta-hospitals.

Munsey, C. (2010). Codd (marble-in-the-neck) soda-water bottles, THEN and NOW! *Historic glass bottle identification and information website*. https://sha.org/bottle/pdffiles/coddarticleMunsey.pdf.

Parramatta Heritage Centre (2015). https://historyandheritage.cityofparramatta.nsw.gov.au/blog/2015/05/26/parramatta-timeline-1788-present.

Rahn, J. (2011). Victorian literature. *The literature network*. http://www.online-literature.com/periods/victorian.php.

Robertson, S. (n.d.) *Nietzsche's critique of morality: a resource for AS-level and A-level philosophy*. Cardiff University. https://www.cardiff.ac.uk/__data/assets/pdf_file/0004/147109/nietzschescritiqueofmorality.pdf.

Sahni, N. (2016). Hugh Taylor – Part 1. Parramatta Heritage Centre, Research Services. https://historyandheritage.cityofparramatta.nsw.gov.au/blog/2016/09/23/hugh-taylor-part-1.

Taylor, D.S. (2000). 1788 – state of the art in textile. *Technology in Australia 1788–1988*. http://www.austehc.unimelb.edu.au/tia/267.html.

References

Newspapers and historical sources

Australian Town and Country Journal 1871–1882

Cootamundra Herald 1889

Cumberland Argus and Fruitgrowers Advocate 1897–1930

Empire 1865

Evening News 1891–1902

Government Gazette 1846–1899

Government Gazette of the State of New South Wales 1904

Historical Records of New South Wales 1892–1914

Illustrated Sydney News 1891

New South Wales Government Gazette 1832–1899

Sydney Gazette and New South Wales Advertiser 1804–1841

Sydney Herald 1836–1841

Sydney Monitor 1834

Sydney Morning Herald 1853–1952

Temperance Advocate and Australasian Commercial and Agricultural Intelligencer 1841

INDEX

ablutions 69, 91
abortion 2, 64
alcohol consumption 26–28, 41, 76–79, 93, 96–98, 101
antiseptic 25, 49, 63, 65, 94
apothecary 40, 41
artefacts 4–5, 17–19, 32–35, 49, 59–60, 61, 68–71, 74–75, 104–114
    aerated water bottles 79–84
    alcohol bottles 76–80
    grooming items 73–75
    medicine bottles 1, 65–68
    schnapps bottles 65–68, 76–80
    tobacco pipes 85–87

barber 40, 72, 94
bathing 25–26, 56, 59, 68–69, 91
benevolent 35–36, 46, 96, 100
bonesetter 40, 62, 63
Burramattagal 7
Byrnes, William 37, 57, 61, 96, 99, 110

case study 4, 5, 14, 17–19, 21, 31, 32–35, 42, 53, 55, 56, 60, 62, 65, 68, 69, 72, 73, 78, 83, 86, 89, 90, 91, 92, 94, 95, 96, 97, 98, 99, 101, 103–114
charity 14, 46, 100
chastity 3, 4, 25, 29, 90, 101
cholera 48, 63, 94
city-wide perspective 1, 17, 89, 101
class structure 1, 3, 21–24, 30, 37, 89, 95, 98
cleanliness 25–26, 68, 73–74, 89, 90–94, 96
convicts 7–9, 12, 14, 21–30, 32, 35–55, 72, 73, 76, 85–86, 89–92, 94, 96, 98–100
culture 1–2, 5, 19, 21–22, 25, 26, 31, 89
Curling, Ellen 36, 64, 94

diphtheria 48, 62–63
discrimination 4, 24, 90, 95, 98–100, 101–102
disease 1, 14, 15, 25, 29, 48–49, 59, 60, 62–63, 65, 85, 90, 91, 94
Dodd, Henry 7–8

environmental reforms 4–5, 18, 39, 41–42, 49, 59–60, 90–91, 101
epidemic 13, 15, 48–49, 60, 61, 90, 94, 100

Female Factory 12, 13, 24, 29, 45, 91–92, 95, 99–100
First Fleet 2, 5, 7–8, 35, 42, 76, 93
friendly societies 2, 14, 15, 40, 46–47, 60

germ theory 8, 48–49, 62, 73, 91, 93–94
gold rush 4, 14, 29, 44
grooming 25, 32, 33, 68–69, 73–75, 87, 91, 92

Hassall, Reverend Rowland 14, 27, 28, 37, 42, 51, 52, 55, 72, 95, 96, 99, 114
health care 1, 4, 5, 7, 9, 14, 39–41, 46, 60, 62, 63, 87, 90, 100, 101, 102
hospital 8, 12, 13, 14, 45–46, 49, 56, 63, 90, 91, 93, 95, 100

Irving, John 7–9

laundry 46, 56, 68, 73–74, 91, 92
Lennox Bridge 8, 13
Lister, Joseph 91

malnutrition 8, 40
Marsden, Reverend Samuel 9, 27, 29, 76
medical anthropology 1, 2, 4–5, 42, 89
medical corps 48, 63, 72
medical practitioner 5, 39–41, 62–64, 85, 87, 93–95, 100
medical reform 28, 94–95, 101
miasma 48
middle class 2, 3, 5, 9, 11, 14, 15, 21, 22–25, 28, 29–30, 31–32, 34–37, 42, 43, 46, 60, 61, 65, 68, 69, 72–74, 76, 85, 86, 89, 91–100, 101–102
midwife 40, 62, 63–64, 94–95
miscarriage 2, 41, 63
Mumford, Mary 3–4

nutrition 12, 39, 40, 42–43, 49, 60, 90, 91

oral hygiene 69, 72, 91–92
orthodox medicine 39, 40, 41, 90, 94–95, 101

Pasteur, Louis 48, 59
pastoralist 5, 13, 22, 24, 30, 43, 44, 89
patent medicine 61, 62, 64–69, 79, 84, 94, 101, 102
personal health 3, 4, 5, 13, 14, 15, 19, 33, 39–43, 60, 61, 63, 73, 87, 90, 101
personal hygiene 1, 4, 26, 33, 49, 61, 68–71, 73, 90, 91
physician 15, 40, 62–64, 100
piety 4, 28–29, 96
plague 25, 48, 63
pollution 26, 52, 53, 56–57, 59, 68, 83, 91
poor 23, 25, 30, 40, 43, 46, 49, 60, 100
Pringle, George 15, 49, 52, 61, 91, 94

quarantine 48, 90

rations 26, 42–43, 85, 93
respectability 1, 3, 4, 5, 25, 32, 39, 46, 84, 86, 87, 90, 92, 93, 95–96, 98, 101–102
Rum corps 3
Rum Rebellion 93

sewerage 15, 18, 49, 52–53, 55, 56, 59, 60, 72, 101
smallpox 12, 15, 48, 63, 94, 101
sobriety 26–28, 101
social reforms 3–5, 18, 19, 21, 26, 28, 33, 61, 76, 85–87, 90, 91, 94, 95, 101
surgeon 2, 3, 7, 8, 12, 13, 15, 21, 36, 40, 42, 43, 48, 49, 62–63, 72, 94

teaware 32, 34–35
temperance 4, 26–27, 30, 65, 76, 79, 83–87, 93–94, 96–98, 101
toys 32–34
traditional medicine 39, 61, 94
tuberculosis 48–49, 63
typhoid 14, 48, 62, 63, 94

vaccination 12, 15, 48, 59, 63, 90, 94
vices 76, 86, 87, 93–94
Victorian values 1, 2–4, 17, 19, 21, 24, 25, 28, 29, 30, 36, 37, 39, 86, 89–90, 95, 96, 98, 101, 102

water supply 4, 9, 14, 15, 17, 18, 49–50, 52–53, 56, 59–60, 68, 83, 84, 90, 91, 101, 108
Wangal clan 7
Wentworth, D'Arcy 11, 14, 21, 36, 96, 108
wise women 62, 94
women's health 63–64, 94